D0984418

COMMON SYMPTOMS OF DISEASE
IN CHILDREN

Common Symptoms of Disease
in Children

R. S. ILLINGWORTH
M.D., F.R.C.P., D.P.H., D.C.H.

Professor of Child Health
The University of Sheffield

FOURTH EDITION

BLACKWELL SCIENTIFIC PUBLICATIONS
OXFORD LONDON EDINBURGH MELBOURNE

ISBN 0 632 09710 8

FIRST PUBLISHED 1967
SECOND EDITION 1969
THIRD EDITION 1971
FOURTH EDITION 1973

Translated into Spanish and Greek

Distributed in the U.S.A. by
F. A. Davis Company, 1915 Arch Street,
Philadelphia, Pennsylvania

Printed and bound in Great Britain by
WILLIAM CLOWES & SONS, LIMITED
LONDON, BECCLES AND COLCHESTER

Contents

vi   *Contents*

Preface to the fourth edition

In preparing this new edition of *Common Symptoms of Disease in Children* I have read and re-read every word of the previous edition and made hundreds of alterations or additions in order to bring it thoroughly up to date. In doing this I have been greatly helped by the criticisms and suggestions of my friends, Dr John Lorber, Dr Victor Dubowitz, Dr Frank Harris and Dr John Black, and have paid careful attention to suggestions made by reviewers of the previous edition. I have not been able to take all the advice offered, because I was most anxious to avoid lengthening the book and making it unwieldy and expensive. One friendly critic advised me to include rashes. On careful consideration I decided not to include them, partly because I am not a dermatologist, and partly because I felt that without illustrations the differential diagnosis would be unsatisfactory: though I have added a short section on different types of rash caused by drugs. I must emphasise that I do not claim that listed causes are in order of importance: it would be impossible to arrange this: but I have tried to point out what conditions I think are rare.

It is very difficult to decide whether to include certain rare diseases. This book is intended not only for family doctors but for other doctors who are faced with a difficult diagnosis of a symptom, and accordingly I have included many rare diseases. Although one is far more likely to be right if one diagnoses the common rather than the rare, an individual child may suffer from a rarity. I have again kept descriptions of conditions, especially rare ones, as brief as possible, because of my constant desire to avoid making the book too big and unwieldy.

Though scores of additions have been made to this volume, by means of extensive pruning and the deletion of repetitions, the book has not been materially lengthened.

Once more I should be most grateful for any suggestions for improving this book in case a further edition is required.

Sheffield, August 1972

Preface to the first edition

When I was talking to my thirteen-year-old child about my attempt to write a book concerning the common symptoms of disease in children, mentioning the difficulties which I was encountering, and the fact that no one, to my knowledge, has attempted it, she said, 'Isn't that all the more reason why you should do it?' I replied that it may well be that the reason why others have not done it is the fact that they had more sense than to try.

I have attempted to write a précis of the common symptoms of disease in children because I felt that the family doctor, when faced with a symptom in a child whom he is examining, would find it useful when in difficulty to refer quickly to conditions which have to be considered. The textbooks, general or specialist, for the most part do not deal with symptoms. For instance, I referred to a large textbook of otorhinolaryngology for information about stridor, but the word was not in the index. It is likely to take a family doctor a long time to find a textbook which discusses the very common cyanotic or apnoeic attacks of the newborn. The great majority of the symptoms which I have discussed in this book are not, in fact, mentioned in the index of the majority of textbooks, and many of the symptoms are not mentioned in the index of any of them. This is not intended to be a criticism of textbooks. Discussion of symptoms would have greatly lengthened them, and inevitably have caused repetition.

In consequence I have discussed about a hundred common symptoms of disease in childhood. I have made no attempt to provide a complete list of all the possible causes of a symptom, but I have tried to pick out the important causes, making it clear which I think are the most common ones, and which I consider to be rare.

Though classifications are useful for memorising, and though they look neat and tidy, I have avoided them almost completely, because of their inherent weakness in not giving the common conditions first.

Where a symptom may be psychological or organic I have included it, but where a symptom is entirely psychological I have omitted it, because I have discussed psychological problems in my books *The Normal Child in His First Five Years** and *The Normal School Child*.† I have, however, included a section concerning psychological manifestations of organic disease, and the somatic manifestations of psychological symptoms.

The book is confined to the subject of diagnosis. I have named common investigations which need to be carried out in order to elucidate the problem—but again have made no effort to name them all. (In a recent article on jaundice in the newborn, the author listed 75 special investigations which should be carried out.) I have not described the normal values of the investigations, nor the methods of performing them: but I have named the investigations in order that the family doctor would know some of the tests which are necessary to establish the diagnosis, and would then know when to refer the child to a special centre for study. I thought, furthermore, that knowledge of the necessary tests would help him in his talks with the parents. I have made a special point of emphasising the conditions which do require such special investigation.

There is inevitably a certain overlap between signs and symptoms and I have allowed myself a little licence in interpreting the word 'symptoms'. For instance, I have included a short section on enlargement of the spleen. Admittedly an adult experiences discomfort when his spleen is felt. My reason for including it, however, was the frequency of splenic enlargement in children and therefore its importance in the diagnosis of so many different diseases.

I have assumed that the family doctor has basic medical knowledge. I have also had to assume that the family doctor does not want or need profound knowledge on any subject. My notes may well, therefore, be criticised for being superficial. They are deliberately made so, because I did not feel that the family doctor would want more. But I have throughout assumed that having looked through a section of this book to read about a particular symptom, he would then refer to one of the recognised textbooks for more

* *The Normal Child*, Fifth Edition, 1972, London, Churchill.
† *The Normal School Child: his problems, physical and emotional*, 1964, London, Heinemann.

information. To this end I have listed principal sources of further knowledge. For instance, as a general source of information on a paediatric problem I have recommended Nelson's *Textbook of Pediatrics*.

In my opinion no one should attempt to make a diagnosis in a sick child without knowing what drugs he has already received. The side effects of drugs are so frequent and far reaching, and the number of drugs taken, whether prescribed by a doctor or otherwise, is so great, that it is essential to know what medicines have been given. I have mentioned the side effects of drugs in the relevant sections, and summarised them in a special section.

At the risk of repetition, I have inserted a brief section about commonly held misbeliefs in paediatric diagnosis—including such a misbelief as the idea that convulsions are caused by teething. I am aware of the fact that there is a small amount of repetition in different sections. I decided to retain this for the convenience of the reader.

I hope that family doctors will find this book useful in General Practice. I believe that students will find this book useful for the purposes of revision. It would not serve as a basic textbook for them, but I believe that it would be useful in conjunction with one of the standard textbooks.

It is certain that many will think of causes of which I have not thought, or of symptoms which should have been included. I should greatly welcome comments and suggestions so that the book can be improved if another edition is required.

I wish to thank my friends Dr Peter Wyon, Family Doctor, of Thirsk, Yorks, Dr Frank Harris, Lecturer in Child Health, the University of Sheffield, and my wife, Dr Cynthia Illingworth, for reading every word of the script and for their most useful criticisms: and to my secretaries, Miss D.Bain, Miss J.Grundy and Mrs D.Ackroyd, for typing the drafts of this book.

Failure to thrive

All those who are concerned with the care of children are repeatedly faced with the problem of the child who refuses to gain weight in the approved manner. It is surprisingly difficult to obtain a composite picture of this problem in the standard texts. In this chapter I have attempted to put together the main conditions which have to be considered when a child's weight gain is below the average. As the problem in the young baby is different from that in the older child, it will be convenient to discuss it in relation to age groupings. In the first place, however, one must decide whether or not there is anything wrong with the child at all.

Variations in normal physical growth

All children are different. Some are small and some are big, some are thin and some are fat. Though nutrition has much to do with this, it is certainly not true to say that nutrition is the only factor. Many factors are unknown. It is always difficult and usually impossible to draw the line between normal and abnormal. A child may be pounds below the average in weight, and inches below the average in height, and yet be perfectly normal. It is far more important that the child should be full of energy, free from lassitude and abounding in *joie de vivre*, than that he should be average in weight and height. One might add that it is much more healthy to be below the average weight than above it. All that one can say is that the further away from the average is the child's weight and height, the less likely it is to be 'normal'.

A child may be unusually small because he takes after his mother or father in that respect. Whenever an infant or older child is unusually small, one should consider the height of the mother and father. A small child, taking after one of his parents in physical build, is not only small in height (or in the case of a baby, in length), but he is less than the average in weight. As a result his appetite is commonly less. The result is that parents are apt to become worried because the child has a smaller intake than usual, and so they try to force him to take more. The inevitable result, after the age of six to nine months or so, is that he refuses. He vomits the food which he is forced to take against his will. He begins to associate mealtimes with tears and unpleasantness, and becomes conditioned against food, so that a troublesome vicious circle and difficult behaviour problem results.

After the first year it is useful to be able to consult a table in order to estimate the child's eventual height. Such a table cannot always

Table 1. Present height in relation to eventual height

(a) *Boys*

	Eventual height		
	5 feet	5 feet 6 inches	6 feet
Age in years	Present height in inches		
1	25·8	28·3	30·9
2	29·4	32·1	35·3
3	31·8	35·1	38·1
4	34·4	37·8	41·2
5	36·6	40·3	43·9
6	38·7	42·7	46·6
7	40·7	44·8	48·9
8	42·6	46·9	51·1
9	44·6	49·0	53·4
10	46·2	50·8	55·5

(b) *Girls*

	5 feet	5 feet 6 inches	6 feet
1	27·0	28·3	32·4
2	31·1	34·3	37·4
3	33·9	37·2	40·6
4	36·5	40·2	43·9
5	39·0	43·0	46·9
6	41·3	45·4	49·6
7	43·5	47·8	52·2
8	45·6	50·1	54·6
9	47·6	52·4	57·1
10	49·5	54·4	59·4

As a rough guide, the height on the second birthday is half the expected adult height. Calculated from Tanner *et al.* (1966). Example—7-year-old girl, height 43·5 inches. Probable eventual height is 5 feet.

be relied upon for accuracy, because so many individual variables
may affect a child's growth; but it may be a good guide which will
help the parent to understand the problem. Tables 2 and 3 show the
average weight and height of British children, while Table 1, based
on the work of Tanner, shows the percentage of eventual height
reached at various ages.

An example of the value of such a table is as follows. A child of
three years was referred because of her small size, being 34 inches

Table 2. Average height of boys and girls

Boys

Age in years	10		50		90		% of adult height
	in	cm	in	cm	in	cm	
0	20·2	51·4	21·3	54·0	22·3	56·6	30·9
1	28·7	72·8	30·0	76·3	31·4	79·7	43·7
2	32·6	82·7	34·2	86·9	35·9	91·1	49·8
3	35·1	89·3	37·1	94·2	39·0	99·1	53·9
4	37·8	96·1	40·0	101·6	42·1	107·1	58·2
5	40·2	102·2	42·6	108·3	45·0	114·4	62·0
6	42·5	108·0	45·1	114·6	47·7	121·2	65·6
7	44·7	113·5	47·4	120·5	50·2	127·5	69·0
8	46·8	118·8	49·7	126·2	52·6	133·5	72·2
9	48·8	124·0	51·8	131·6	54·8	139·3	75·4
10	50·7	128·8	53·9	136·8	57·0	144·8	78·3

Girls

Age in years	10		50		90		% of adult height
	in	cm	in	cm	in	cm	
0	19·8	50·4	20·9	53·0	21·9	55·6	32·7
1	27·9	70·8	29·2	74·2	30·6	77·7	45·7
2	32·0	81·3	33·7	85·6	35·4	89·8	52·8
3	34·7	88·1	36·6	93·0	38·5	97·9	57·3
4	37·4	94·9	39·5	100·4	41·7	105·9	61·9
5	39·8	101·1	42·4	107·2	44·6	113·2	66·1
6	42·0	106·8	44·5	113·4	47·2	120·0	69·9
7	44·2	112·4	47·0	119·3	49·7	126·3	73·6
8	46·3	117·6	49·2	125·0	52·1	132·4	77·1
9	48·4	122·9	51·4	130·6	54·4	138·3	80·5
10	50·5	128·3	53·7	136·4	56·9	144·5	83·8

high. Her mother was five feet tall and was relieved to hear that the girl could be expected to reach the same height as she had.

Table 3. Average weight of boys and girls

Boys

Age in years	10		50		90	
	lb	kg	lb	kg	lb	kg
0	6·17	2·8	7·72	3·5	9·04	4·1
0·25	11·05	5·01	13·07	5·93	15·41	6·99
0·5	14·99	6·8	17·42	7·9	20·28	9·2
0·75	17·59	7·98	20·28	9·2	23·43	10·63
1·0	19·40	8·8	22·49	10·2	25·79	11·7
2	24·25	11·0	28·0	12·7	32·19	14·6
3	28·00	12·7	32·41	14·7	37·26	16·9
4	31·52	14·3	36·60	16·6	42·11	19·1
5	34·61	15·7	40·72	18·5	47·4	21·5
6	38·14	17·3	45·20	20·5	52·91	24·0
7	41·89	19·0	49·82	22·6	59·29	26·9
8	46·03	20·9	55·11	25·0	66·13	30·0
9	50·48	22·9	60·62	27·5	73·63	33·4
10	55·56	25·2	66·80	30·3	82·23	37·3

Girls

Age in years	10		50		90	
	lb	kg	lb	kg	lb	kg
0	6·28	2·85	7·50	3·4	8·71	3·95
0·25	10·6	4·81	12·26	5·56	14·13	6·41
0·5	14·2	6·44	15·21	6·9	18·72	8·49
0·75	16·71	7·58	19·22	8·72	22·09	10·02
1·0	18·52	8·4	21·38	9·7	24·69	11·2
2	22·93	10·4	26·89	12·2	31·09	14·1
3	27·11	12·3	31·52	14·3	36·15	16·4
4	31·09	14·1	35·93	16·3	41·44	18·8
5	35·05	15·9	40·34	18·3	47·17	21·4
6	38·8	17·6	44·97	20·4	53·79	24·4
7	42·33	19·2	49·82	22·6	61·07	27·7
8	46·29	21·0	55·34	25·1	68·78	31·2
9	50·7	23·0	61·07	27·7	78·04	35·4
10	55·34	25·1	68·56	31·1	90·39	41·0

Tanner, J.M., Whitehouse, R.H., Takaishi, M. (1966). 'Standard from Birth to Maturity for Height, Weight, Height Velocity and Weight Velocity.' *Arch. Dis. Childh.*, **41**, 613.

The next most common factor to consider when an apparently well child is unusually small for his age is the birth weight, and in particular the birth weight in relation to the duration of gestation. The smaller the child is at birth, the smaller he is likely to be in later years, and the larger he is at birth, the larger is he likely to be in later childhood. There is evidence that the baby who is small at birth in relation to the duration of pregnancy is likely to be even smaller in later years than the child whose weight at birth corresponded with the usual weight for the duration of gestation. It seems as if the child's growth potential was indicated by his unusually small growth in utero, and that his subsequent growth is correspondingly less than that of most other children (Illingworth, 1972).

Many mothers are worried about the normal slowing down of the weight gain in the second half of the first year. This is associated with a falling off in the appetite. It is apt to cause food forcing and so food refusal. Others are worried by the small appetite of a child who has a small build because he takes after the mother or father or has congenital heart disease or other condition which affects physical growth. Once more, this is apt to lead to food forcing and so to food refusal. It is important that parents should know that children take all that they need if given a chance, and that it is never necessary to try to make a child eat. A poor appetite in a well child is always due to food forcing. A poor appetite is most unlikely to cause defective nutrition.

Defective physical growth from previous disease, now cured

There is evidence from work on animals that if growth is retarded in early life, the growth remains defective later in spite of adequate nutrition.

Many human infants who suffered major surgical procedures in the early weeks, and who were excessively small in weight in that period, are small in later years. (Eid. 1970.) The longer the growth retardation persisted before the cause is corrected, the greater is the subsequent growth deficit. Umansky & Hauck (1962) showed that children operated on for ligation of a patent ductus arteriosus, and who were far below the average in size at the time of the operation, did not usually catch up to the average height after the ligation. In fact only 20 per cent of 444 children showed a marked postoperative acceleration of growth in height. It seems that there is a 'critical period' in physical growth, and that after that a normal diet will not restore the child to an average size.

For true dwarfism, see p. 20.

Other causes to consider

The following is a useful classification of the causes of failure to thrive:

Defective intake
  Breast feeding without weight checks
  Artificial feeding
    Fear of overfeeding
    Errors in preparing the feeds
    Incorrect feeding of premature baby
    Inadequate fluid in hot climates
  Emotional deprivation; prolonged crying; child abuse
  Chronic infection, e.g., urinary tract
  Vitamin deficiency on synthetic diets
  Subdural haematoma (rare)
  Pink disease (rare)
Defective Absorption
  Fat. Steatorrhoea, including fibrocystic disease of the pancreas, coeliac disease, and other conditions
  Carbohydrate. Carbohydrate intolerance
  Protein
  Hirschsprung's disease
Increased loss
  Excessive perspiration. Overclothing
  Vomiting
  Diarrhoea
Errors of metabolism (all rare)
  Renal acidosis
  Hypercalcaemia
  Nephrogenic diabetes insipidus
  Adrenocortical hyperplasia
  Hypophosphatasia

Organ diseases, involving the brain, heart, chest, kidney, liver, pancreas
  Mental deficiency, cerebral tumour, subdural haematoma
  Congenital heart disease
  Severe asthma, bronchiectasis, tuberculosis
  Chronic renal insufficiency
  Cirrhosis of the liver
  Diabetes mellitus
Chronic infection
No known cause

Defective intake

A breast-fed baby is more likely to suffer from underfeeding than an artifically fed baby, because the mother cannot know how much milk she has without weighing the baby. In my experience every mother thinks that the leaking of milk from the breast (lactorrhoea) signifies that there is an abundance of milk, though it signifies nothing more than the draught reflex, or the unusually easy escape of milk from the breast. Many doctors think that if a baby is contented he must be obtaining sufficient milk from the breast. This is far from the truth. Many young babies are content to starve and do not cry, even though they are receiving a totally inadequate amount of milk.

The most accurate way of establishing the diagnosis of defective intake in a breast fed baby is the test feed—weighing the baby before and after every feed in the day, expressing milk fully after each feed and measuring it, and then adding up the total. If expression is not carried out, the result is seriously misleading, for all that one is then measuring is the milk which the baby has taken from the breast, but not the milk available in the breast. If a baby sucks badly or is drowsy or irritable or if the nipple is a difficult one for him, he may not obtain milk which is in the breast.

An artificially fed baby may be underfed either because of starvation, or because of *errors in the constitution of the feeds*. In investigating the method of feeding, it is essential to ask how much milk powder, sugar, and water the mother is putting into each feed. It is futile to accept a mother's statement that she is giving the baby 'five ounces of Cow and Gate' at each feed. She may be making the feed up far too dilute, so that the baby is underfed.

One of the commonest causes of underfeeding is the *fear of over-feeding*. Mothers wrongly ascribe the vomiting, the loose stools, the crying or the wind to overfeeding, when in fact they are due to underfeeding. They then reduce the quantities taken and starve the baby still further. Overfeeding may interfere with weight gain in a small premature baby because of fat intolerance, but not in a full term baby, who knows when to stop.

In hot climates I have seen infants who were given quantities of fluid suitable for the British climate, but unsuitable for the country in question. They were being given 2½ ounces per pound (160 ml per kg) per day, which is the usual quantity needed in England, but insufficient in a country such as Egypt, where there is more fluid loss through perspiration.

A small premature baby may refuse to gain weight on human milk, but thrive on skimmed cow's milk. A common cause of the failure of a premature baby to gain weight is inadequate intake: it is commonly forgotten that whereas a full term baby usually needs 2½ ounces of milk per pound per day (160 ml per kg), a prema-ture baby after two weeks usually needs 3 ounces per lb per day (188 ml per kg) and 4 ounces per lb per day (250 ml per kg) after four weeks: but overfeeding may cause vomiting and loss of weight.

When a baby is seriously underweight, one commonly finds that the quantity which the mother states that she is giving is adequate, but that when the baby is admitted to the ward he is ravenously hungry, has a far bigger than average weight gain, and has been half starved. I have known such babies gain as much as 25 ounces a week when given as much as they want. *It is important to accept with scepticism the mother's story of the quantity given. When a child is failing to thrive, and no obvious cause can be found, one should suspect underfeeding, whatever the mother says.*

In the case of the older infant and young child, underfeeding may be due to parental food fads and ignorance.

An important cause of defective intake of food is *emotional de-privation*. One often sees older babies who refuse to gain weight in hospital, in the absence of evidence of disease. They gain weight normally when the mother is admitted to the hospital to be with the child, or when she takes him home. An important cause of failure to thrive is excessive crying. There are many possible causes of this (p. 239). Continual crying not only uses up energy, but also leads to loss of fluid through the lungs and so causes defective weight gain. It may also tire the baby, so that when food is offered he does not take it well.

Child abuse, often termed the battered baby syndrome, is an example of severe emotional deprivation. It may take the form of emotional cruelty, deliberate starvation, the deprivation of fluid, physical trauma (broken bones, bruises, subdural haematoma, the infliction of burns, injury to the mouth or viscera), or the administration of poison or overdose of drugs. As child abuse is always denied by the parents, diagnosis can be difficult. Factors which should arouse suspicion are repeated injuries, complaints about the child's bad behaviour and delay in calling for medical help.

Chronic infection, such as that of the urinary tract, may prevent a satisfactory weight gain.

Mann, Wilson & Clayton (1965) described *deficiency states in infants on synthetic foods* (e.g., low phenylalanine for phenylketonuria, low lactose for galactosaemia, low sodium and low calcium). The children failed to thrive and developed sores around the external nares, fissured lips, lesions at the outer canthus of the eyes, angular stomatitis and psoriasiform lesions on the buttocks. They responded immediately to Ketovite tablets and syrup.

For reasons which we do not altogether understand, a chronic *subdural haematoma* in an infant may cause failure to thrive. It may act through reduction of the appetite or by causing vomiting.

Pink disease, due to mercury intoxication, causes defective intake and failure to thrive.

Before embarking on the many complex investigations for failure to thrive, involving errors of absorption, metabolism and increased loss of nutriments, it is essential to be sure that the cause is not a simple matter of defective intake. This is not always easy to eliminate.

Defective absorption

When considering the cause of failure to thrive due to defective absorption, one must think of defective absorption of fat, carbohydrate and protein.

Defective absorption of fat (steatorrhoea)

There are many causes of steatorrhoea (Di Sant'Agnese and Jones (1972)). In an analysis of 266 cases of steatorrhoea in children, Charlotte Anderson found that 52 per cent were due to fibrocystic disease of the pancreas, 35 per cent to coeliac disease, and 13 per cent to other causes, of which the main ones were giardiasis, chronic intestinal infection, anomalies of the alimentary tract, and certain diseases of the liver and pancreas.

The commonest cause of steatorrhoea is *fibrocystic disease of the pancreas.* It occurs in approximately one in every 2400 children. There are four main modes of presentation—meconium ileus in the newborn baby, failure to thrive, steatorrhoea, and chronic or recurrent chest disease. Meconium ileus (p. 64) presents as intestinal obstruction in the newborn. Failure to thrive is seen at any age in young children from infancy onwards. Bulky, offensive or loose stools may be noticed by the mother at any stage, but this is relatively unusual. In many cases of coeliac disease or fibrocystic disease of the pancreas, the mother has not noticed anything unusual about the stools. One should always investigate for fibrocystic disease when a child has chronic pulmonary infection such as bronchiectasis or persistent radiological abnormality in the lung such as pulmonary collapse. One does not suspect fibrocystic disease merely because the child develops a cough whenever he has a cold. Two other signs may draw attention to the possibility of fibrocystic disease—unexplained generalised oedema or prolapse of the rectum. There are other causes of both of these conditions, but both are sometimes early features of steatorrhoea and in particular fibrocystic disease of the pancreas. Cirrhosis of the liver is sometimes a feature of fibrocystic disease of the pancreas.

The diagnosis of fibrocystic disease is established by the demonstration of steatorrhoea by a fat balance test or measuring the fat output, and by estimation of the salt content of the sweat. Stools are collected for a minimum of five days; over the age of 18 months, a fat output of over 4 g per day or an absorption of less than 90 per cent is abnormal. Below the age of 18 months an absorption of less than 85 per cent of the intake is abnormal.

It is wrong to think that one can eliminate the possibility of steatorrhoea by inspecting the stools. Stools which prove to contain a significant excess of fat may look completely normal. The diagnosis of steatorrhoea cannot be made by inspection of the stools or by microscopic examination. It must be made by a fat balance or by measuring the fat output.

Coeliac disease is the second most common cause of steatorrhoea. The majority of cases are due to sensitivity to gluten, but a few may be due to milk allergy. It should be noted that many examples of so-called milk allergy have recently been shown to be due not to allergy to milk protein, but to carbohydrate intolerance. Disaccharide intolerance may be associated with coeliac disease; the child as a result does not do well on a gluten-free diet until lactose and sucrose are also excluded.

The symptoms of coeliac disease commence when cereals are introduced into the diet, so that the age of onset is variable. The usual initial symptom is vomiting. Other symptoms are undue irritability, loss of appetite and failure to thrive. In an advanced case there is wasting of the buttocks with a protuberant abdomen (as in other forms of steatorrhoea). The appetite in coeliac disease tends to be poor, while that in fibrocystic disease tends to be unusually good, but in the absence of chronic pulmonary infection one cannot distinguish the two conditions on clinical grounds. The diagnosis of coeliac disease is confirmed by the demonstration of steatorrhoea by estimation of the faecal fat output, with normal sweat sodium, by jejunal biopsy and barium meal. It is wrong to base the diagnosis on the therapeutic test, if this can be avoided, because once one has embarked on the special diet it is difficult to discontinue it because of fear of harming the baby. In severe cases six to eight weeks may elapse before improvement occurs.

Steatorrhoea may result from *chronic intestinal infection*, particularly by *giardiasis* or *salmonella*. Fresh warm stools should be examined for giardiasis, but duodenal intubation may be required for detection of vegetative forms. Though rare in England, giardiasis is common in many developing countries.

Certain *congenital anomalies of the alimentary tract* may cause steatorrhoea. They include *malrotation, stenosis, gastrocolic fistula, intestinal lymphangiectasia* and *intestinal reduplication* (Leslie & Matheson, 1965). *Crohn's disease* (regional ileitis) may cause failure to thrive due to defective absorption of protein and fat. There may be no other symptom or sign pointing to that condition (Sobel *et al.*, 1962). More often there is abdominal pain and sometimes a low-grade fever. The clinical diagnosis would be confirmed by finding a mass in the right iliac fossa, particularly if there were a sinus. Unusual symptoms include clubbing of the fingers, polyarthritis, iridocyclitis and anal fistulas.

There is an association of steatorrhoea with *pancreatic insufficiency and chronic neutropenia.*

Steatorrhoea may be found in cases of *carbohydrate intolerance, anaphylactoid purpura, protein losing enteropathy* (p. 14), *tuberculosis of the mesentery, biliary atresia* and *cirrhosis of the liver*. There may be some steatorrhoea in conjunction with *ulcerative colitis*. It is found in the rare a-beta-lipoproteinaemia in which there is ataxia, absence of beta-lipoproteins in the serum, reduced serum lipoids and a crenated appearance of the red cells (acanthocytosis). Retinal changes occur in the later stages.

Steatorrhoea may result from the administration of certain *drugs* —neomycin, kanamycin, paromomycin and P.A.S.

Carbohydrate intolerance and malabsorption

A variety of carbohydrate enzyme defects have been described in the last few years. Some of them are genetically determined, while others are secondary to conditions involving the alimentary tract, such as coeliac disease, fibrocystic disease of the pancreas, sprue, gastroenteritis and giardiasis. They should be seriously considered whenever one is faced with the problem of a child with failure to thrive and loose stools. The stools are tested for reducing substances by the Clinitest, and if that is positive, the sugar is identified by paper chromatography. When the Clinitest is performed, the child must be on a normal diet.

Lactose intolerance presents usually with diarrhoea, vomiting, lactosuria and failure to thrive. Symptoms begin as soon as the baby is put to the breast. The child promptly improves when lactose is excluded from the diet. The diagnosis is confirmed by the presence of sugar in the stools, lactosuria and the lactose tolerance test.

In *alactasia* there is diarrhoea due to unabsorbed disaccharides, because of defective absorption of lactose. The child improves when sucrose is given and lactose is excluded. The Clinitest on the stools is positive.

Maltose or *sucrose intolerance* are rather less common. Diarrhoea and failure to thrive are the usual features.

Fructosaemia has been the subject of many papers (Levin *et al.*, 1965). There is vomiting, failure to thrive, lassitude, perspiration, trembling, palpitation and fits, with hepatic enlargement and sometimes jaundice. Some of the symptoms are the result of hypoglycaemia. The symptoms begin when the child eats sugar, sweets, fruit, honey or certain vegetables. There are no symptoms when the baby is breast feeding. There may be albumin and fructose in the urine and abnormal animo-aciduria. There may be a particular aversion to sweet foods. There is usually no diarrhoea. The symptom of fits on eating sugar suggests the diagnosis. The Clinitest on the stools is positive. The diagnosis is confirmed by a fructose tolerance test, in which the blood fructose and glucose are estimated after a standard dose of fructose. The fructose rises while the glucose falls.

Amylase deficiency is associated with diarrhoea.

Galactosaemia usually presents in the newborn baby with vomiting, purpura, weight loss, and jaundice with hepatic enlargement, as soon as he receives breast milk. Cataracts and mental deficiency soon develop. Galactose is found in the urine. The Clinitest or Benedict test is positive. The Clinistix may also be positive, because the damaged renal tubule allows glucose to leak through. The diagnosis is confirmed by the galactose 1 phosphate uridyl transferase estimation in the red cells.

Defective protein absorption

This may be due to chronic diarrhoea from any cause, such as ulcerative colitis. It may be due to deficiency of trypsinogen

(Townes, 1965); this presents with oedema due to hypoproteinaemia. Duodenal intubation and nitrogen balance studies demonstrate the deficiency of trypsinogen.

The so-called exudative enteropathy is a condition in which there is generalised oedema due to protein loss in the stools. It may result from ulcerative colitis, regional ileitis or other conditions. There is a low serum albumin and gamma globulin, and a positive polyvinyl-pyrrolidone test.

Hirschsprung's disease

Defective absorption and failure to thrive may result from Hirschsprung's disease. There will be a history of severe constipation from birth, often with abdominal distension, and a story that no stool was passed in the first 24 to 36 hours. On the other hand the symptom of constipation may not be impressive, and the diagnosis may be missed because of attacks of severe diarrhoea and vomiting. These suggest gastroenteritis, when in fact the cause is Hirschsprung's disease. On rectal examination it is found that the rectum is empty. The diagnosis is confirmed by means of a barium enema and rectal biopsy for deficiency of ganglion cells.

Increased loss of nutriments and fluid

Excess loss of fluid in perspiration may result from *over-clothing or an excessively hot environment*. It leads to constipation and failure to gain weight adequately. The loss of fluid through the lungs resulting from excessive crying has already been mentioned.

Chronic vomiting or diarrhoea will prevent an adequate weight gain.

Some metabolic causes of failure to thrive

When a baby or toddler who is failing to thrive in spite of adequate food intake is found to be grossly constipated, one should think of one of the conditions associated with polyuria, notably renal acidosis, hypercalcaemia and particularly in a boy, nephrogenic diabetes insipidus.

Renal tubular acidosis is an uncommon but important condition of infancy. It is important because appropriate treatment will enable the baby to gain weight normally, and failure to diagnose it is likely to lead to the child's death. It is manifested by vomiting and failure to thrive, often with polyuria. It seems to be due to failure of the renal tubules to reabsorb bicarbonate. The diagnosis is made by simultaneous estimation of the plasma bicarbonate and the urinary pH. There is acidosis in the blood and an alkaline or insufficiently acid urine.

Idiopathic hypercalcaemia presents with similar symptoms. There is polyuria with resulting constipation. In severe cases there is a characteristic facies and a systolic cardiac murmur. The diagnosis is made by estimation of the serum calcium. Proper treatment may prevent mental deterioration and should enable the child to thrive normally.

Nephrogenic diabetes insipidus is another condition with symptoms like those of renal acidosis. The diagnosis can usually be established by the finding of a high serum sodium, a high urea nitrogen and a fixed low specific gravity in the urine. Tests are needed to distinguish it from diabetes insipidus due to pituitary deficiency, and investigation in hospital is essential.

Adrenocortical hyperplasia with salt loss may cause vomiting, diarrhoea and failure to thrive. The diagnosis would be suggested when a girl is found to have a large clitoris or a boy has a large penis—though the enlargement of the penis may not be obvious. The presence of hypospadias in an infant who is not thriving would immediately suggest the likelihood that the child is a girl with virilisation due to adrenocortical hyperplasia. Pigmentation of the nipples and scrotum is a useful sign in affected boys. The buccal smear should establish the nuclear sex. Estimation of the plasma electrolytes is needed, with estimation of the urinary 17 ketosteroids and pregnantriol. It is urgent to make the diagnosis, for many affected babies die in early infancy without the diagnosis being made, whereas they would have survived with proper treatment.

Hypophosphatasia. Children with this rare condition fail to thrive, have rickets, other bone deficiencies, and sometimes vomiting, constipation and convulsions.

Organ disease involving the brain, heart, chest, kidney, liver or pancreas

A variety of diseases of the brain, heart, chest, kidney, liver and pancreas may be responsible for the failure of the infant to thrive. *Certain brain diseases*, other than mental deficiency, are associated with defective physical growth. *Mentally defective children*, especially when they also have cerebral palsy, are commonly malnourished, partly because they are unable to chew until much later than a normal child. As a result they have to be fed on semi-liquid feeds, and defective intake of necessary foodstuffs may result. In such children it is easy to miss the age at which the child learns to chew, and if he is not given solids at the time when he has recently learnt to chew, he will be diffident about taking them later, refusing them or vomiting. This depends on the so-called 'sensitive' or 'critical period' (Illingworth & Lister, 1964). Defective physical growth in mentally defective children may be due to the underlying brain defect.

A *craniopharyngeal cyst* may cause defective physical growth. I have seen children with this condition who presented with defective weight gain and no other symptoms. Ophthalmoscopic examination may point to the diagnosis. The finding of unilateral optic atrophy or of papilloedema would point to the need for further investigation, including an x-ray of the skull for ballooning of the sella or calcification.

Other *neoplasms in the region of the hypothalamus and third ventricle, including the diencephalic syndrome*, are associated with failure to thrive. Affected children are emaciated, notably alert, and have a normal or increased appetite. The onset is usually in the first year. After a period of accelerated growth, loss of weight occurs. There may be signs of autonomic disturbance, such as profuse sweating, and there may be nystagmus. There are usually no abnormal neurological signs and there is no papilloedema. The important feature in many is a high C.S.F. protein. Pituitary function tests may show evidence of pituitary deficiency.

Subdural haematoma has already been mentioned.

Congenital heart disease, such as a patent ductus arteriosus, atrial or ventricular septal defects, or Fallot's tetralogy, is usually asso-

ciated with stunting of growth. The reasons for this are not altogether clear. I have seen several examples of severe food refusal
resulting from food forcing, which in turn resulted from the
parents' anxiety about slow weight gain and smallness of size in
children with congenital heart disease. It is important that the
cause of the stunting of growth should be recognised, partly because
it may be remedied surgically, and partly because the parents may
then avoid food forcing.

Bronchiectasis, asthma and other chronic pulmonary conditions
are likely to be associated with defective weight gain. Most children
with severe asthma are small in height and below the average
weight. This is aggravated by prolonged corticosteroid treatment.
Tuberculosis in England is now a rare cause of failure to thrive.

Renal insufficiency should be remembered when an infant or
child is not thriving. It may be due to congenital renal fibrosis,
polycystic kidneys, hydronephrosis or chronic pyelonephritis. A
clean specimen of urine should be examined for the specific gravity,
albumin or sugar and for the deposit and culture. The importance of the specific gravity is commonly forgotten. A fixed low
specific gravity suggests renal insufficiency or other cause of polyuria. The blood urea and blood pressure should be recorded.

It should not be difficult to diagnose *cirrhosis of the liver*, a rare
cause of failure to thrive. One cause of cirrhosis of the liver is fibrocystic disease of the pancreas. Other causes include hepatolenticular
degeneration, diagnosed largely by the estimation of serum copper
oxidase and tyrosinosis, which is associated with renal tubular defects and rickets (Halvorsen *et al.*, 1966).

Diabetes mellitus will be readily eliminated by examination of
the urine. Fibrocystic disease of the pancreas is discussed elsewhere.

Chronic infection

Acute infections, even when frequent, do not usually cause defective weight gain, because children have a compensatory increase of
appetite after a febrile illness and make up lost ground, but a severe
chronic infection such as bronchiectasis or urinary tract infection
may well cause defective weight gain.

Congenital cytomegalovirus or toxoplasma infection may lead to failure to thrive. There may be hepatosplenomegaly and purpura with retinal changes.

Summary of the principal investigations required to elucidate defective weight gain

The main parts of the clinical examination which are apt to be forgotten, and which are relevant to establishment of the diagnosis, are the examination of the optic fundi, the blood pressure and of the urine especially for the specific gravity. The urine must also be examined for albumin, reducing substances and the deposit (for infection), and it must be cultured. It may also have to be examined for abnormal aminoaciduria. The plasma bicarbonate and urinary pH must be examined simultaneously for evidence of renal acidosis. Other investigations include in particular the serum electrolytes and calcium, the blood urea, fat balance, jejunal biopsy, sweat test, and examination for carbohydrate intolerance.

There are many more investigations which may be needed for the elucidation of the particular problem, but the above are the main investigations needed.

Conclusion

Provided that the family doctor has satisfied himself that the unduly small infant or small child is not small merely because he takes after one of his parents, or because he was an unusually small baby at birth, and that the problem is not merely one of defective intake, he should have the problem investigated by an expert. The problem of failure to thrive is one of the most difficult and yet one of the most common problems facing the paediatric physician. It is important to make the diagnosis in order that the appropriate treatment can be given. Failure to do so may mean that the child will not survive or that his growth will remain permanently defective.

References

ADDY D.P. & HUDSON F.P. (1972) Diencephalic syndrome of infantile emaciation. *Arch. Dis. Childh.*, **47**, 338.

ANDERSON C.M., TOWNLEY R., FREEMAN M. & JOHANSEN P. (1961) Unusual causes of steatorrhoea in infancy and childhood. *Med. J. Aust.*, **2**, 617.

BAIN H.W., DARTE J.M.M., KEITH W.S. & KRUYFF E. (1966) The diencephalic syndrome of early infancy, due to silent brain tumour, with special reference to treatment. *Pediat.*, **38**, 473.

CORNBLATH M. & SCHWARTZ R. (1966) *Disorders of Carbohydrate Metabolism in Infancy.* Philadelphia, Saunders.

DI SANT' AGNESE P. & JONES W.O. (1962) The coeliac syndrome (malabsorption) in pediatrics. *J. Am. Med. Ass.*, **180**, 308.

EID E.E. (1970) A follow up study of physical growth following failure to thrive with special reference to a critical period in the first year of life. *Acta Paediat. Scandinavica.* In press.

EID E.E. (1970) Studies on the subsequent growth of children who had retardation and acceleration of growth in early life. Ph.D. Thesis, University of Sheffield.

HOLZEL A. (1967) Sugar malabsorption due to deficiencies of disaccharidase activities and monosaccharide transport. *Arch. Dis. Childh.*, **42**, 341.

HUBBLE D. Disorders in growth, in Gairdner D. (1965) *Recent Advances in Paediatrics.* London, Churchill.

ILLINGWORTH R.S. (1972) *The Normal Child.* London, Churchill Livingstone.

ILLINGWORTH R.S. & LISTER J. (1964) The critical or sensitive period with special reference to certain feeding problems in infants and children. *J. Pediat.*, **65**, 839.

LESLIE J.W.M. & MATHESON W.J. (1965) Failure to thrive in early infancy due to abnormalities of rotation of the mid-gut. *Clin. Pediat.*, **4**, 681.

MANN T.P., WILSON M. & CLAYTON B.E. (1965) A deficiency state arising in infants on synthetic foods. *Arch. Dis. Childh.*, **40**, 364.

SMITH D.W. (1967) Compendium on shortness of stature. *J. Pediat.*, **70**, 463–519.

SOBEL E.H., SILVERMAN F.L. & LEE C.M. (1962) Regional ileitis without symptoms. *Am. J. Dis. Child.*, **103**, 575.

TANNER J.M., WHITEHOUSE R.H. & TAKAISHI M. (1966) Standard from birth to maturity for height, weight, height velocity and weight velocity. *Arch. Dis. Childh.*, **41**, 613.

TOWNES F.L. (1965) Trypsinogen deficiency disease. *J. Pediat.*, **66**, 275.

UMANSKY R. & HAUCK A.J. (1962) Factors in growth of children with patent ductus arteriosus. *Pediatrics*, **30**, 540.

Dwarfism

True dwarfism in a child is rare, and in this section I do not propose to discuss in detail the various causes, because it is of little importance in the practice of the family doctor. It may present diagnostic difficulties in infancy if the body proportions are normal.

The principal causes are:

(i) Skeletal diseases. The commonest of these are achondroplasia and vitamin D resistant rickets.

(ii) Endocrine diseases. These include hypopituitarism, thyroid deficiency, pseudohypoparathyroidism, adrenal disease (e.g. Cushing's syndrome), and in a girl, gonadal dysgenesis.

(iii) Chromosomal abnormalities, e.g. Turner's syndrome, testicular feminisation.

(iv) Drugs.

Achondroplasia should be readily diagnosed by the short humerus and femur. When the child puts his hands down by his side, it is obvious that they do not reach as far as those of a normal child. Most children with this condition have a large head, due either to hydrocephalus or to megalencephaly, with a depressed bridge of the nose. There are several rare allied conditions.

Vitamin D resistant rickets is commonly familial. If the child is walking, there is usually bowing of the legs. The diagnosis of rickets is confirmed by x-ray of the wrists and estimation of the serum calcium, phosphorus and alkaline phosphatase.

Hypopituitarism is rare in children. The child is usually dwarfed but of normal proportions. The diagnosis can only be established by investigations which include an x-ray of skull (for the pituitary fossa), growth hormone and other pituitary hormone assays.

A child with *thyroid deficiency* is small in height because of delayed skeletal maturation. He retains the infantile proportions of a longer upper than lower segment (pubis to heel). One should think of this diagnosis when a child stops growing before puberty. The infant with thyroid deficiency has the characteristic facies of

20

the cretin, but when an older child develops thyroid deficiency the facies may not be characteristic. The diagnosis is established for an x-ray for skeletal maturation, the protein bound iodine and the estimation of the total serum lipoids.

Pseudohypoparathyroidism is a rare condition in which there is shortness of stature, short fingers and often mental subnormality and fits. The middle finger may be shorter than the index finger. There is a low serum calcium. Various laboratory tests are required to establish the diagnosis.

For *Cushing's disease* see p. 26.

Turner's syndrome in girls is diagnosed in infancy by the finding of oedema of the lower limbs, often with webbing of the neck, pigmented naevi, coarctation of the aorta, a low hair line at the back of the neck, cubitus valgus and a short fourth metacarpal. Later there is small stature and absence of secondary sexual characteristics. It is easy to diagnose cubitus valgus when it is non-existent. Usually when the upper arms are fully extended and touching, the forearms cannot without difficulty be brought parallel, whereas they can in Turner's syndrome (and some normal people). The short fourth metacarpal is demonstrated by placing a ruler or firm card across the outer knuckles: normally the ruler will not touch all three knuckles. If there is a short fourth metacarpal, the card touches the third and fifth metacarpals, acting as a bridge over the fourth. The diagnosis of Turner's syndrome is confirmed by a buccal smear, chromosome analysis and biochemical tests. There are variants of Turner's syndrome which in the older child are less easy to diagnose; the height may be normal or increased and the appearance of the child may be normal, apart from the absence of breast enlargement. The urinary gonadotrophins would be raised and the vaginal smear is a useful test.

The child with the *Prader-Willi syndrome* has commonly a low birth weight, sucking difficulties in early infancy, small height, small hands and feet, undescended testes, a hypoplastic scrotum, hypotonia in the early months, and subsequently by the second or third year, obesity. The child is dwarfed, and diabetes may develop later.

Corticosteroids given in large dosage for a long time cause severe stunting of growth.

The method of investigating dwarfism was discussed by Gordon (1971).

Reference

GORDON R.R. (1971) Endocrine disorders in adolescence. *Practitioner*, **206**, 189.

Loss of weight

When a child loses weight, other than in the course of an acute infection, one always feels concern. There are many possible causes, some of them serious.

In considering a mother's complaint that the child has lost weight, the first essential is to determine the evidence for her statement. Usually she has no figures to support her claim, but she may say that the child's clothes no longer fit because they are now too big for him. The child has been weighed on different scales—perhaps one time in clothes and another time without—and the mother had not thought of the possibility that the scales were inaccurate. When the weight of a baby is to be compared one day with that at another, it is essential that it should be recorded on each occasion at the same time in relation to feeds. It would not be profitable to weigh the baby before a feed one day and to compare his weight after a feed on another day.

Loss of weight, other than that during an ordinary acute infection such as gastroenteritis, may be due to any of the following conditions, amongst others:

Emotional causes

Conditions causing persistent vomiting

Conditions causing diarrhoea

Conditions associated with polyuria
  Diabetes mellitus
  Diabetes insipidus
  Hypercalcaemia
  Renal acidosis
  Renal failure

Malabsorption
  Fats (steatorrhoea)
  Carbohydrates (intolerance)
  Protein
  Hirschsprung's disease

Pink disease

Infections
  Urinary tract
  Tuberculosis
  Partial collapse of the lungs
  Other

Rheumatoid arthritis

Asthma

Drugs

Rarely—thyrotoxicosis, Addison's disease, malignant disease, muscular dystrophy

In the section 'Failure to Thrive' it was stated that an infant separated from his mother may fail to gain weight, or may lose weight. Worries about home or school may cause an older child to lose weight. I have seen anorexia nervosa in older children who have been teased on account of obesity.

Persistent vomiting, such as that due to hiatus hernia, or *persistent diarrhoea*, as in ulcerative colitis, may cause loss of weight.

A useful test which should always be carried out when there is unexplained loss of weight is estimation of the specific gravity of the urine. A fixed low specific gravity would lead to investigation for one of the causes of *polyuria*, such as renal failure, nephrogenic diabetes insipidus or hypercalcaemia. Diabetes mellitus must be eliminated by testing the urine for reducing substances. The other causes of polyuria have been described in the section entitled 'Failure to thrive'.

Loss of weight may be due to *malabsorption*, including fibrocystic disease of the pancreas and coeliac disease. In the case of carbohydrate intolerance there is usually some diarrhoea.

Pink disease should no longer be seen, now that mercury is no longer included in teething powder, but mercury can be given in other ways, and Pink disease should not be regarded purely as a disease of the past.

A chronic *urinary tract infection* may present as loss of weight with lassitude. No examination of a child who has lost weight is complete without microscopy and culture of a clean specimen of urine. In the same way no examination would be complete without a tuberculin test unless the child has previously been given BCG.

Lassitude and loss of weight following what appeared to be a simple upper respiratory tract infection may be due to *partial collapse of the lungs*. This may be suspected because of physical signs, but an x-ray is needed for confirmation.

The vagueness of the symptoms of the pre-arthritic stage of *rheumatoid arthritis* is mentioned in the section on unexplained fever.

Most children with *severe asthma* are underweight and some lose weight.

Certain *drugs* may cause loss of weight. When one institutes treatment for cretinism with thyroxin, some loss of weight is common. It is said that loss of weight may be a side effect of sulthiame.

Thyrotoxicosis and *Addison's disease* are rare in children, but the signs are the same as those in adults and can hardly be missed.

Malignant disease, whether cerebral, intra-thoracic, intra-abdominal or elsewhere, may be the cause of loss of weight.

There is general muscle wasting in the later stages of *muscular dystrophy*.

Generalised *lipodystrophy* is a rare cause of loss of weight. The child will be well, and it can be seen that the appearance of emaciation and the weight loss are due to loss of fatty tissue only.

Conclusion

Loss of weight is one of the important symptoms of childhood which demands full investigation, except where the cause is obvious, such as gastroenteritis or diabetes mellitus. Hospital laboratory facilities are usually necessary for the elucidation of this symptom. Loss of weight is a symptom which must never be taken lightly.

Excessive height

The following are the usual causes of excessive height:

Heredity
Cerebral gigantism
Additional Y chromosome
Marfan's syndrome

The commonest reason for excessive height is genetic—the child taking after one of his parents. Obese children are usually tall for their age (until the epiphyses fuse). Children with precocious puberty or adrenocortical hyperplasia are tall for their age.

Cerebral gigantism is rare. It is associated with mental deficiency, an odd face (often hypertelorism), antimongoloid slant of the eyes, prognathism and fits.

An additional Y chromosome is often associated with tallness and a tendency to delinquency.

Marfan's syndrome of arachnodactyly, dislocation of the lens and congenital heart disease is associated with excessive height.

Reference

OTT J.E. & ROBINSON A. (1969) Cerebral gigantism. *Am. J. Dis. Child.*, **117**, 357.

Obesity

The commonest type of obesity is the so-called *simple obesity*—a misnomer, because the cause of all obesity is far from simple. Basically this is due to an imbalance between intake and output, the child eating more than he needs. Most fat children have developed the sweet-eating habit, and are commonly to be seen eating potato crisps, lollipops and ice creams, large quantities of sugar in their drinks and frequent glasses of orange squash.

Mothers argue that the children are so big that they need a lot to fill them; and that they have a 'marvellous appetite'. There are often important emotional factors which cause overeating. A useful review is that of Jean Mayer (1966). Obesity in the early weeks, shown by Eid to be related to obesity in later years (1970), may be due to the premature administration of cereals.

Obesity may develop because of inactivity—as in prolonged bed rest, the Werdnig–Hoffmann syndrome, muscular dystrophy in its later stages, mongolism or severe cerebral palsy especially around puberty. It may be responsible for severe respiratory symptoms (the Pickwickian syndrome). A rare cause of obesity is the *adenoma of the islet cells of the pancreas* causing hypoglycaemia and hunger. *Corticosteroids* cause obesity.

Most fat children are tall for their age because of secondary adrenocortical overactivity, but their epiphyses fuse prematurely so that most of them are ultimately small.

If a fat child is small for his age, the following conditions should be considered:

Cushing's syndrome.
Prader-Willi syndrome (p. 21).
Turner's syndrome (p. 21).
Thyroid deficiency (p. 20).
Pituitary syndromes.

In *Cushing's syndrome* there is a characteristic distribution of fat, involving mainly the trunk (buffalo hump) and face, with relatively normal limbs: a plethoric face with red cheeks, a deep voice, hypertrichosis, purple striae and often hypertension. Tests for adrenal function include estimation of the 17 ketosteroids, 17 hydroxyketosteroids, measurement of the diurnal rhythm of plasma cortisol, urinary free cortisol and the dexamethazone test. The presence of striae in a fat child should not lead one to diagnose Cushing's disease, for striae occur normally in fat children.

The *pituitary syndromes* are extremely rare. Frölich's syndrome is so rare that I have not yet seen a case. It consists of obesity, dwarfism, hypogonadism, optic atrophy, headache, polyuria and glycosuria, due to a cyst in the region of the pituitary. The apparent smallness of the penis should not lead one to the erroneous diagnosis of Frölich's syndrome: the penis is buried in the fatty tissue and looks smaller than it really is. The Laurence Moon Biedl syndrome consists of obesity, polydactyly, retinitis pigmentosa, mental subnormality and hypogonadism.

Not all small fat children fall into the above categories: the relatively small height cannot always be explained.

References

CAYLER G.C., MAYS J., RILEY H.D. (1961) Cardiorespiratory syndrome of Obesity (Pickwickian Syndrome) in children. *Pediatrics,* **27,** 237.

EID E.E. (1970) Follow up study of physical growth of children who had experienced excessive weight gain in the first six months of life. *Brit. Med. J.,* **2,** 74.

JOURNAL OF THE AMERICAN MEDICAL ASSOCIATION (1970) Obesity: a continuing enigma. Leading Article. **211,** 492.

MAYER J. (1966) Some aspects of food intake and obesity. *New Engl. J. Med.,* **274,** 662, 722.

WIDDOWSON E. (1970) Harmony of growth. *Lancet,* **1,** 901.

Unexplained fever

In this section I shall refer to the problem of prolonged temperature elevation whose cause has not been determined by taking the history and examining the child—there being no abnormal physical signs apart from the fever and the appearance of illness. It is assumed that the physical examination has included the inspection of the eardrum for otitis media. The problem is a fairly common one, and it is one which it may be extremely difficult to solve even with the fullest laboratory assistance.

The following conditions should be considered, not necessarily in the order of likelihood:

Normal variation
Dehydration
Absorption of blood. The effect of trauma and surgical procedures
Malingering
Infections

Rheumatoid arthritis (pre-arthritic stage)
The effect of drugs and poisons
Rare causes—
  Collagen diseases
  Reticuloses and malignant disease
  Alimentary conditions
    ulcerative colitis
    regional ileitis
  Liver disease
  Subdural haematoma
  Ectodermal dysplasia
  Caffey's disease
  Agammaglobulinaemia
  Familial dysautonomia

Normal variations

Excitement or exertion may cause a slight rise of temperature. The temperature should not be taken immediately after a hot drink.

Bakwin (1944) described five infants with what he called 'psychogenic fever'. They had a persistent low grade fever when in hospital separated from their mothers, and the temperature fell to normal as soon as they went home.

An occasional child has a slight persistent elevation of the temperature, or a daily elevation up to 38°C, without any discoverable disease. The elevation of temperature is usually discovered after some childhood infectious disease or tonsillitis. The child appears to be well and is symptom-free. Exhaustive tests fail to reveal any abnormality. Eventually the parent is advised to stop taking the temperature, and on follow-up study the child remains well. These cases are always worrying and have to be investigated and followed up with the greatest of care, but one never feels confident in the conclusion that there is no disease. One would be especially uncertain if the child, in addition to the elevation of temperature, does not feel well, energetic and free from lassitude, or if his weight gain is not satisfactory. A good non-specific test which helps, and one which is easily carried out in the doctor's surgery, is the ESR. A normal figure does not exclude disease but it does make it less likely. A raised figure does mean that disease is present and must be looked for.

It must be remembered that a rectal temperature is commonly a little higher than that in the mouth. The rectal temperature depends on the depth to which the thermometer is inserted. Those interested should read the excellent monograph written by Talbot many years ago (Talbot, 1931).

Dehydration

The so-called *dehydration fever of the newborn* consists of a sudden rise of temperature a day or two after birth. It is thought to be due to loss of fluid. The temperature rapidly settles when boiled water or other fluid is given.

Any baby may develop a rise of temperature if overheated. The most striking example of this occurred during a ward round. A baby was well when I saw him, but an hour later had a temperature of 41°C and was severely dehydrated, because his crib had been in contact with a radiator. The dehydration was such that he had to be given an immediate intravenous infusion.

Because of the absence of sweat glands, the temperature may rise in infants with *ectodermal dysplasia* when overheated. In the congenital anhydrotic type of ectodermal dysplasia, the child seems to be normal at birth. Later there is a dry skin, unexplained fever, sparse hair, delayed or absent dentition or widely space incisors and conical canines, often with a saddle shaped nose and frontal bossing. In the dominant hydrotic form there are dystrophic nails, hyperkeratosis of the palms and soles, absent or sparse hair at birth, and later hypertrichosis and pigmentation.

A rise of temperature may result from other conditions causing dehydration, apart from the ordinary infections. These include *nephrogenic diabetes insipidus* and *idiopathic hypercalcaemia*.

Absorption of blood—trauma, surgical procedures

The rise of temperature under these circumstances is only short lived, and should not cause confusion in the diagnosis for more than a day or two.

Malingering

I have seen serious diagnostic difficulties from malingering in child-hood. A ten-year-old girl was referred from another hospital on account of high swinging fever of some weeks' duration. She had been extensively investigated and no cause had been found. The suddenness of the rise of temperature and the fact that the girl was well when the temperature was markedly raised suggested the diagnosis of malingering. When a nurse turned her back she rapidly rubbed the bulb of the thermometer with her bedclothes. Vigorous rubbing of the bulb of the thermometer will raise the mercury from 36°–40° C in some five seconds. It takes longer to raise the temperature to that point by placing it in contact with the average hot water bottle.

Urinary tract infection

The most common cause of fever in a child without abnormal physical signs is a urinary tract infection. There are usually no symptoms referable to the urinary system, and it is not usual to find either loin tenderness or albumin in the urine.

The absence of infection in a specimen of urine does not absolutely exclude a serious infection. The flow of urine from a pyonephrosis may be blocked, the urine examined having come from the other kidney.

For notes on the method of collecting a specimen of urine, see p. 264.

Other infections

Tuberculosis can be eliminated by a tuberculin test. If a child has miliary or meningeal tuberculosis, however, the tuberculin test may be negative on account of anergy. On ophthalmoscopic examination choroidal tubercles can be found in over 60 per cent of children with miliary tuberculosis. An x-ray of the chest would clinch the diagnosis. Meningeal tuberculosis would be confirmed by lumbar puncture. In all other forms of tuberculosis the tuberculin test would be positive. Investigations necessary include x-ray of the chest, microscopy of the urine for tubercle bacilli and culture or guinea pig inoculation of stomach washings.

In *typhoid and paratyphoid fever* there is almost always enlargement of the spleen, and there are usually rose spots on the abdomen. The diagnosis is established by blood culture and possibly by agglutination reactions.

Brucellosis is rarely seen in Britain. It is usually accompanied by fever and an enlarged spleen. The diagnosis is established by agglutination reactions and blood culture.

Roseola infantum can cause confusion for three or four days. The child has a high temperature for that period without abnormal physical signs, and then the temperature subsides as the erythematous rash develops.

An occasional child may have a raised temperature throughout the incubation period of *measles*. In many other children there is a high temperature for five or six days, in association with an infection of the upper respiratory tract, before the measles rash appears. Koplik's spots can be seen in the buccal mucosa during the pre-eruptive phase.

Infectious mononucleosis (glandular fever) may occasionally present with fever but without other abnormal signs, though there is usually enlargement of the spleen and often lymph node enlargement. The diagnosis is made by the finding of abnormal lymphocytes in the blood smear, the Paul Bunnell reaction and the rapid Monospot slide test.

Acute toxoplasmosis and *acute cytomegalovirus infection* resemble glandular fever. The diagnosis would be confirmed by serological tests.

Toxocara canis or catis infection may give no abnormal signs apart from fever. It is diagnosed by skin and agglutination tests.

Meningococcal septicaemia may present as fever of unknown origin. It is essential to look carefully for petechial haemorrhages, particularly on the conjunctival surfaces of the eyelids. A joint effusion in conjunction with petechiae would suggest the diagnosis and a blood culture would confirm it.

Certain *closed-off abscesses* may give rise to fever without physical signs, at least for a time. They include particularly the subphrenic or perinephric abscess, a pulmonary abscess or an abscess in a silent area of the brain. The pulmonary abscess can be seen in an x-ray of the chest, but the others may present difficulty. Continued fever following an attack of abdominal pain should suggest the possibility of a subphrenic abscess following the perforation of an appendix. An x-ray may show gas under the diaphragm. A perinephric abscess may present considerable difficulties. It may be preceded by trauma or a staphylococcal skin infection. There are likely to be rigors, and there may be pain on the affected side, with pain on flexing the spine. There are not usually urinary symptoms. An x-ray may show a bulging psoas shadow. There is usually intermittent but not continuous pyuria.

A cerebral abscess is usually associated with headache and often with neck stiffness. There is often but not always papilloedema, but there may be no localising neurological signs. The diagnosis would be suspected if there had been a neighbouring focus of infection, as in the ear or scalp, or if there were bronchiectasis or congenital heart disease. It would be confirmed by lumbar puncture, echogram, electroencephalograms, scanning and air studies. A cerebral abscess may persist undiagnosed for some weeks. In the case of all these abscesses, with the occasional exception of the cerebral abscess, the white cell count is likely to show a polymorphonuclear leucocytosis, and the erythrocyte sedimentation rate (esr) would probably be raised.

A low grade *osteitis* may cause considerable difficulty in diagnosis. The possibility must be remembered in any child with prolonged low grade fever and signs of an infection. The routine examination of any child with unexplained fever must include palpation of all the bones for local tenderness, and if there is a suspicion of tenderness (or if there is local pain), an x-ray should be taken. I have known a low grade osteitis persist for many months before localising signs developed. A raised esr and a polymorphonuclear leucocytosis should suggest the possibility. A blood culture should always be taken.

A child with unexplained fever without abnormal physical signs may have a low grade *septicaemia*. If there is a heart murmur, the possibility of subacute bacterial endocarditis should be remembered. A particularly careful search for petechiae should be made, and the urine should be examined for excess of red cells in the deposit.

An *apical tooth infection* may cause difficulty in diagnosis. We have seen several examples of such infection in children receiving corticosteroids. The infection was painless and there were no local signs pointing to the root of the tooth. When a child or adult has an unexplained fever (or lassitude), the teeth should be examined. If any tooth is known to be dead, an x-ray of the tooth should be taken.

When children have lived in countries in which amoebic infections occur, an *amoebic abscess of liver* should be considered. There may (or may not be) obvious liver enlargement. There is a polymorphonuclear leucocytosis. Screening may show decreased movement of the diaphragm on the affected side. Sigmoidoscopy may show amoebic ulcers and amoebae may be found in the stools.

Subclinical hepatitis may cause unexplained fever. A history of exposure to infection, together with liver function tests may lead to the correct diagnosis.

Rheumatoid arthritis

This may present as prolonged fever without arthritis (p. 227).

The reticuloses and collagen diseases

Systemic lupus erythematosus, dermatomyositis and periarteritis nodosa must be considered when there is unexplained fever.

Systemic lupus may present with fever, a butterfly rash on the face, arthralgia and thrombocytopenic purpura. There may be polyserositis, hepatosplenomegaly, enlarged nymph nodes, hypertension and albuminuria. There may be puncta on the palms and fingertips. The blood should be examined for LE cells. It may follow the use of a variety of drugs, including carbamazepine, ethosuccimide, griseofulvin, isoniazid, 6 mercaptopurine, P.A.S., penicillin, phensuccimide, phenytoin, primidone, streptomycin, sulphonamides, tetracycline, thiouracil and troxidone.

Periarteritis nodosa can be present with unexplained fever. One should palpate the skin of the whole body for nodules, which consist of aneurismal dilatations of the vessel walls. There is often albuminuria and leucocytosis with eosinophilia. The diagnosis is confirmed by biopsy.

In *Hodgkin's* disease and *the reticuloses*, splenic enlargement is usually present. Unless there is obvious lymph node enlargement, permitting biopsy, the diagnosis can be difficult. There is often a hypoplastic anaemia, sometimes with considerable leucocytosis. Sometimes a bone marrow examination reveals the nature of the condition.

Alimentary conditions

Ulcerative colitis may be associated with fever, but the presence of diarrhoea with blood and mucus in the stools usually points to the diagnosis. *Regional ileitis* can cause fever with failure to thrive for some weeks before alimentary symptoms develop.

Liver disease

Cirrhosis of the liver, malignant tumours and other conditions of the liver including subclinical hepatitis may be associated with fever.

Drugs

The so-called drug fever, which occurs especially with sulphonamides, but occasionally with other antibiotics, including rifampicin, may cause considerable difficulty in diagnosis. The temperature falls by crisis when the drug is withdrawn. Other drugs may sometimes cause elevation of the temperature. They include acetazolamide, amphetamines, azathioprine, cephalosporins, colistin, meprobamate, methimazole, nitrofurantoin, nortriptyline, P.A.S. and thiouracil. Certain drugs in an overdose may cause a rise of temperature. They include antihistamines, drugs of the atropine group and mono-amine oxidase inhibitors.

Miscellaneous

A *subdural haematoma* in an infant may be accompanied by fever. The fontanelle may be bulging and there are likely to be retinal haemorrhages.

Hereditary ectodermal dysplasia may be associated with fever from the early days of life. The dry skin and later the dental condition should reveal the diagnosis.

Caffey's disease in the newborn baby may be manifested by unexplained fever for 3 or 4 weeks before the characteristic swelling of the jaw and perhaps tender swellings of the tibiae, due to periostitis, become obvious.

Agammaglobulinaemia and *Riley's syndrome* of *familial dysautonomia* may be associated with unexplained fever.

Summary of special investigations needed for the elucidation of unexplained fever

Urine microscopy and culture
Complete blood count, sometimes with bone marrow examination. Search for LE cells
ESR
Paul Bunnell reaction for infectious mononucleosis. Monospot slide test
Tuberculin test. Where necessary, culture and guinea-pig inoculation of stomach washings
Culture of faeces
Blood culture
Agglutination reactions—salmonella, brucellosis, toxocara (with skin test)
X-ray chest, and where indicated bones, or x-ray of abdomen. Pyelogram where indicated
Liver function tests
Wassermann reaction
Electrophoresis—serum proteins
Where indicated, barium meal and follow through
X-ray of the jaw for Caffey's disease

References

BAKWIN H. (1944) Psychogenic fever in infants. *Am. J. Dis. Child.*, **67**, 176.
BITNUN S., DAESCHNER C.W., TRAVIS L., DODGE W. & HOPPS R. (1964) Dermatomyositis. *J. Pediat.*, **64**, 100.
JACOBS J.C. (1963) Systemic lupus erythematosus in childhood. *Pediatrics*, **32**, 257.

ROBERTS F.B. & FETTERMAN G.H. (1963) Polyarteritis nodosa in infancy. *J. Pediat.*, 63, 519.

SHEON R.P. & VAN OMMEN R.A. (1963) Fever of obscure origin. *Am. J. Dis. Child.*, 34, 486.

TALBOT F. (1931) Skin temperatures in children. *Am. J. Dis. Child.*, 42, 965.

Lassitude

It is common to hear the complaint that a child seems to be constantly tired or lacking in energy. In this section only chronic lassitude will be discussed. Lassitude of acute onset is likely to be due to an infection, such as measles or tonsillitis.

The following are conditions which have to be considered when there is chronic lassitude or lack of energy:

Developmental feature
Insufficient sleep
Puberty
Psychological factors, including personality and insecurity
Familial feature
Hypoglycaemia
Anaemia
Low grade infection, such as pyelonephritis, tuberculosis
Persistent haemolytic streptococcal throat infection, or early rheumatic fever
Apical tooth infection
Partial collapse of the lung
Rheumatoid arthritis
Effect of drugs
Rarely
    Myasthenia gravis
    Dermatomyositis
    Muscular dystrophy
    Gilbert's disease
    Subacute bacterial endocarditis
    Addison's disease

Apparent lack of energy may be a *developmental feature*. It is common for a child of two to five or so to show little inclination to play outside and to seem to become tired too easily.

After infancy lassitude may be due simply to *insufficient sleep*. Children may go to bed too late or stay awake for a long time—usually as a result of mismanagement by the parents.

Many mothers become worried when the boy or girl at *puberty* seems to have no energy after having been constantly 'on the go' only a year or two previously. This is a common feature of early puberty. Nevertheless, it is the doctor's responsibility to see that there is not one of the other causes, such as tuberculosis, anaemia or a urinary tract infection.

Many children are thought to be lacking in energy and easily tired when the problem is entirely a matter of their *personality*, which is usually a familial feature. Some children prefer to read books rather than to play active games out of doors: some prefer their own company and that of their family to that of children in the street. Sometimes children are afraid of going out to play or are worried about so doing, because they are teased by others or are being bullied. A child may seem to his mother to be tired and lacking in energy when he is well and fit but worried about home or school, or feeling insecure. It may also be a feature of boredom.

A child may refuse to play with others and therefore prefer to stay indoors because he is a *'clumsy'* child (p. 172), and cannot keep up with other children. His mother may think that he is tired or lacking in energy.

One must never conclude that a child's lassitude is entirely psychological until one has eliminated organic disease, because organic disease may cause behaviour problems. Lassitude, pallor and irritability before meals may be due to *hypoglycaemia*.

Low-grade anaemia is an important organic cause of lack of energy and easy fatigability. If there is any doubt a haemoglobin estimation should be performed.

A common cause of undue fatigue and vague unwellness is a chronic *urinary tract infection* (p. 264). It is essential to eliminate a tuberculous infection by performing a Heaf tuberculin test.

One commonly sees children who are well until they develop acute tonsillitis, and are then tired and lacking in energy for three or four weeks or more. This may be due to a *persistent haemolytic streptococcal infection*, or may represent the onset of an attack of rheumatic fever. It is worth while taking a throat swab and carrying out a therapeutic test with oral penicillin for ten days, provided that other causes have been eliminated.

Whenever there is unexplained fatigue (or unexplained fever), an *apical tooth infection* should be considered, especially if it is known that there is a dead tooth. An x-ray examination is required.

Another infection not infrequently seen in a children's hospital out-patient departmental is *partial collapse of the lungs*. The child presents with lassitude and perhaps a slight cough, following a respiratory infection without known pneumonia. The clinical signs may suggest the diagnosis, but an x-ray photograph of the chest is required to establish it.

A useful non-specific test for children with undue fatigue is the ESR. If it is normal, it does not eliminate organic disease; but if it is raised, it makes organic disease certain, and an infection is the most likely cause.

Rheumatoid arthritis may present as easy fatigability and sometimes with unexplained fever for weeks or months before eventually arthritis becomes manifest (p. 226).

Drugs may give rise to the complaint of lassitude. This may be due to drowsiness or to muscle weakness. Muscle weakness may be a side effect of amitryptyline, chloroquin, ethosuccimide, nalidixic acid, piperazine or streptomycin. Corticosteroids may cause weakness through a form of myopathy.

Rare causes of the symptom of lassitude include *myasthenia gravis, dermatomyositis, Gilbert's disease, muscular dystrophy*, and *subacute bacterial endocarditis*.

Myasthenia gravis is rare in childhood. The symptoms become more marked towards the end of the day. The first symptom may be ptosis. The child may find it tiring to climb stairs or to walk. There is no atrophy of muscle. The therapeutic test with neostigmine is valuable confirmatory evidence. Electromyography and other tests should be carried out.

Dermatomyositis may be present as fatigue and weakness, especially in the legs. The child is miserable, and the muscles may feel stiff. There may be a facial rash with a violaceous hue, periorbital oedema and characteristic 'cigarette paper' lesions on the knuckles, elbows and knees. The skin tends to become bound to the underlying tissues at the joints. It occurs at any age including infancy. It is more common in girls than boys.

Gilbert's disease is rare. It consists of a mild low-grade persistent jaundice. *Subacute bacterial endocarditis* would be suspected if there were a congenital or acquired heart disease.

Muscular dystrophy may present as easy fatigability. The child cannot walk far, and in the Duchenne type finds it difficult to get up stairs. The serum creatine phosphokinase will help to establish the diagnosis when there is doubt.

References

SIMPSON J.A., Myasthenia gravis, in WALTON J. (1964) *Disorders of Voluntary Muscle*. London, Churchill.

Excessive sweating

Causes of excessive sweating other than that due merely to a hot environment, include the following:

Fever
Over-clothing
Emotional factors
Thyrotoxicosis and thyroxin overdosage
Pink disease
Familiar dysautonomia (Riley's syndrome)
Effect of drugs

Sweating hands are often a feature of normal children and adults.

Sweating around the head in bed is often a notable feature in normal children. It is an ill understood symptom, which used to be ascribed to rickets, and which is not associated with any particular disease.

Fever of any cause may lead to excessive sweating, and

over-clothing is a common cause of the symptom. Many babies are grossly over-clothed in warm or cold weather, and I have seen severe sweat rashes, including 'prickly heat' in such children.

Children with a certain emotional make-up may sweat excessively.

Pink disease, due to mercury intoxication, may be a cause of excessive sweating.

The symptom may be due to amitriptyline, amphetamine, antihistamines, ephedrine, imipramine, pethidine and the phenothiazines.

Attacks of excessive sweating may be associated with the following conditions:

(a) Vasomotor disturbance, such as fainting, especially if there is anaemia, or if there were recumbency due to illness.
(b) Hypoglycaemia (rare).
(c) Pain (such as abdominal colic).
(d) Rarely—phaeochromocytoma, neuroblastoma.

If there are unexplained attacks of excessive sweating not associated with fainting, one should consider *hypoglycaemia, phaeochromocytoma* or *neuroblastoma*. Hypoglycaemia is diagnosed in the first place by a fasting blood sugar. Phaeochromocytoma causes attacks of headache, sweating, fits, pallor, polydipsia, vomiting and lassitude, is associated with hypertension, and is diagnosed by a variety of tests, including estimation of the urinary output of noradrenaline and its metabolites.

Pulmonary tuberculosis in childhood is an exceedingly rare cause of night sweats. To put it in another way, night sweats do not suggest the diagnosis of pulmonary tuberculosis in young children.

Excessive sweating is one of the symptoms of *Riley's syndrome* of familial dysautonomia (rare). The child does not shed tears. He sweats excessively, has a blotchy rash and exhibits hypotonia and areflexia. There is a characteristic smooth tongue without the normal papillae. The affected newborn baby usually has difficulty in sucking and swallowing, has poor muscle tone, and an absent or poor Moro reflex. The condition is usually associated with mental subnormality. Riley's syndrome is a genetic condition with an error of catecholamine metabolism. In the urine there is an excess of products of catecholamines, such as homovanillic acid.

Reference

FREEDMAN A.R. (1966) Familial dysautonomia. *Clinical Pediatrics*, **5**, 265.
VOORHEES M.L. (1966) Functioning neural tumours. *Pediatric Clinics N. America*, **13**, 3.

Enlargement of the lymph nodes

The important causes of enlargement of the lymph nodes in children are the following:

Infection
> Cervical nodes—tonsillitis, other throat infection, scalp and other skin conditions. Infectious mononucleosis. Primary tuberculosis. Rubella

Axillary
> Sore areas on the skin of the arm
> Result of BCG or smallpox vaccination

Inguinal
> Sore places on the skin of the lower limb
> Perianal or other perineal infection

General
> Infectious mononucleosis. Toxoplasmosis, cytomegalovirus
> Tuberculosis, syphilis. Serum sickness
> Brucellosis, tularaemia. Infection from scratching (e.g. eczema). Leukaemia. Reticuloses and neoplasms.
> Cat scratch fever (rare).

Drug—phenytoin.

The commonest cause of enlargement of the lymph nodes is *infection*. Those in the neck are enlarged if there is infection in the throat, in the skin of the face, the skin behind the ear or the scalp. When there is no other obvious source of infection, one must examine the scalp for sore places in association with pediculosis or other infection. Regional lymph nodes may be enlarged as a result of a small and apparently insignificant skin lesion due to primary tuberculosis. Black & Chapman (1964) described children with cervical adenitis due to organisms which resembled the tubercle bacillus. Many similar cases have been described in different parts of the world.

In the case of enlargement of the axillary lymph nodes, the cause may lie in *BCG or smallpox vaccination*.

Almost all persons have palpable inguinal lymph nodes. They are commonly said to be enlarged when they are normal. It is easy to forget to examine the perianal region when the nodes are enlarged.

In *infectious mononucleosis* there is not necessarily enlargement of the nodes. In most children only the cervical ones are involved. There are clinical conditions which closely resemble infectious mononucleosis but in which the usual tests for that infection are persistently negative. Toxoplasmosis and cytomegalovirus infection give a similar picture, and can be diagnosed by serological tests. *Tuberculosis* may cause general lymph node involvement.

Cat scratch fever is due to a virus infection. Ten to thirty days after infection there is malaise, fever and enlargement of the lymph nodes draining the infected area. Keratitis and encephalitis have sometimes occurred as complications. The diagnosis may be confirmed by an intradermal skin test.

Other causes include *serum sickness* (after an antitoxin), *leukaemia, Hodgkin's disease*, and other *reticuloses* and *neoplasms*.

Various *drugs* may cause lymphadenopathy. They include cephaloridine, iron dextran, meprobamate, P.A.S., phensuccimide, phenylbutazone, primidone, sulphadimine and troxidone. Phenytoin may cause not only lymphadenopathy but also hepatosplenomegaly.

Investigations needed include a full blood count, a Paul Bunnell test, a throat swab in the case of cervical adenitis, a therapeutic test of pencillin when in doubt about a streptococcal cause of cervical adenitis, tests for toxoplasmosis and cytomegalovirus, and when all else fails to give the answer, and if the enlargement is significant, a biopsy for histological examination. One must not wait too long before carrying out a biopsy, because of the importance of instituting treatment early in the reticuloses.

Reference

BLACK R.G. & CHAPMAN S. (1964) Cervical adenitis in children due to human and unclassified mycobacteria. *Pediatrics*, **33**, 887.

Anaemia and pallor

Many children are treated for anaemia in family practice when in fact there is no anaemia at all. The child may be pale because he has been indoors a great deal, is tired, or has an infection, or because he has a pale complexion, taking after a parent in that respect. In mild degrees of anaemia it is impossible to be certain of the diagnosis without a haemoglobin estimation.

Many are unaware of the normal levels of haemoglobin at different ages. The following are normal figures in grammes per cent (O'Brien and Pearson, 1971).

	Mean	Range
Cord blood	17·1	13·7–20·5
7 days	18·8	14·6–23·0
20 days	15·9	11·3–20·5
45 days	12·7	9·5–15·9
75 days	11·4	9·6–13·2
120 days	11·9	9·9–13·9
1 year	12·2	10·0–13·0
5 years	12·5	12–13
10 years	13·5	13–14
Older	15	14–16

The normal range in the young baby depends on the birth weight. A drop from 16·0 g at birth to 8·0 g at 6 weeks is normal for a 1·5 kg low birthweight baby, but not at 2 weeks, and is not normal for a full term baby.

In the newborn baby, the usual cause of anaemia at birth is haemolytic anaemia due to blood group incompatibility; but it could be due to bleeding from a placental vessel, foeto-maternal transfusion, or in the case of twins, to bleeding of one twin into the other. An important cause is bleeding from the umbilical cord, whose ligature has become slack with contraction of the cord; and on the second to about the fifth day, the most likely cause is blood loss due to haemorrhagic disease of the newborn. Anaemia may arise in the first few days as the result of infections.

In later infancy the most likely cause is prematurity. It is by far the commonest cause of anaemia between six and 12 months of age. Another cause is severe anaemia in the mother in the latter part of pregnancy. From ten months onwards nutritional anaemia is the most common, due to a poor diet.

A simple classification of the causes of anaemia is as follows:

Blood loss
Nutritional defects
Infection
Haemolysis
Defective red cell production and other serious blood diseases

Anaemia due to blood loss

Bleeding from placental vessels, or into the placental circulation
Bleeding of one twin into the other
Bleeding from the umbilical cord
Haemorrhagic disease of the newborn
   Melaena. Haematemesis
Extensive cephalhaematoma
Nose bleeds
Bleeding from the alimentary tract
   Oesophageal varices
   Hiatus hernia
   Aspirin and other drugs
   Hookworms
   Haemangioma
   Meckel's diverticulum (pp. 86, 107)
   Reduplication of intestine (p. 86)
   Telangiectasia (p. 86)
   Ulcerative colitis (pp. 82, 86)
   Rectal polyp (p. 86)

Bleeding from the urinary tract
Blood diseases—haemophilia, etc
Trauma

Bleeding from placental vessels, etc. This is the second most common cause of anaemia at birth, the most common being haemolytic disease of the newborn. It is due to rupture of the cord, anomalous placental vessels, damage to the placenta by instruments or separation of the placenta. Transplacental haemorrhage may also occur; this consists of bleeding into the maternal circulation. The child is pale and the pallor persists in spite of normal respirations and the administration of oxygen. It is important to note that the child's pulse is rapid, while the child with pallor due to anoxia has a slow pulse. If the haemoglobin is below 9 grammes per cent, transfusion is urgent.

Bleeding of one twin into the other. One twin is born plethoric, the other anaemic. Both twins may need treatment, the plethoric one needing a replacement transfusion, replacing some blood by plasma, and the other needing the administration of blood.

Bleeding from the umbilical cord. Bleeding from the umbilical cord is usually due to contraction of the cord, leaving the ligature slack. Serious bleeding may occur and an urgent transfusion may be required.

Haemorrhagic disease of the newborn. When a newborn baby in the first three or four days vomits blood or passes blood per rectum, it is essential to determine whether it is the mother's blood, swallowed during delivery or from her nipple, or the baby's blood, because if it is the baby's blood, the appropriate treatment must be given (usually Vitamin K) and a careful watch must be kept in order to determine whether a transfusion is necessary. The material should be filtered, and to 5 parts of the supernatant fluid one adds 1 part of 0·25 N (1 per cent) NaOH. If the colour changes to yellow, it is the mother's blood, and if it remains pink, it is the baby's blood, because the foetal haemoglobin is more resistant to alkali. This condition is a matter of urgency. It is a tragedy to allow an infant to die from melaena neonatorum when his life could readily have been saved by a transfusion.

It is rare for bleeding into a *cephalhaematoma* to be excessive. If it does occur, it should suggest a blood disease such as haemophilia. It is common for haemophilia to occur without a family history of that condition.

Oesophageal varices are likely to be found only in cases of cirrhosis of the liver or hypersplenism.

Hiatus hernia is an important cause of bleeding. The diagnosis should be suspected when an infant or child has a long history of vomiting, with occasional traces of blood in the vomitus. The diagnosis may be established by a barium swallow and faecal occult blood tests.

Aspirin may cause gastric bleeding, and if given frequently, may cause severe anaemia. The bleeding occurs largely as a result of direct irritation of the mucosa of the stomach by particles of aspirin, and it may also be due to hypoprothrombinaemia or thrombocytopenia. Various *other drugs* may cause gastrointestinal haemorrhage. They include acetazolamide, antimetabolites, chlortetracycline, indomethacin and thiazides. Intestinal bleeding may also be caused by methotrexate, and by thiazides administered with potassium chloride.

Hookworm infection is an important cause of anaemia due to blood loss in tropical countries or in immigrants from those countries. The diagnosis is made by the finding of ova in the stools.

Meckel's diverticulum, reduplication of the intestine, ulcerative colitis and rectal polyp are discussed on pages 86 and 107. For other causes of blood in the stool, see p. 84.

Haematuria. Prolonged haematuria may follow an attack of acute nephritis. I have seen severe anaemia develop from this cause.

Haemolysis

Haemolytic disease of the newborn
   Blood group incompatibility, including ABO incompatibility
Acholuric jaundice; spherocytosis
Hereditary nonspherocytic haemolytic anaemia
Sickle cell anaemia
Cooley's anaemia (thalassaemia)
Glucose 6 phosphate dehydrogenase deficiency
Pyruvate kinase deficiency

Autoimmune haemolytic anaemia
Drugs
Infections
Acute haemolytic anaemia of unknown origin
Haemolytic uraemic syndrome
Periarteritis and disseminated lupus

This list is by no means complete, but it does include the more important conditions.

The most common cause of anaemia on the first day of life is *haemolytic disease*, and this is almost certainly the diagnosis if in addition there is jaundice. The possibility of prenatal blood loss must be remembered. *As treatment may be urgently needed, it is vital that an exact diagnosis should be established immediately, with the help of the Blood Transfusion Laboratory or other laboratory service.* The Coombs' test in ABO incompatibility is commonly negative.

Acholuric jaundice. A family history of acholuric jaundice or unexplained anaemia should alert one to the diagnosis. The spleen is almost always enlarged. The diagnosis is established by the spherocytosis in the blood film, the reticulocytosis and increased red cell fragility. There is a rare hereditary nonspherocytic haemolytic anaemia.

Sickle cell anaemia. There are several types of sickle cell anaemia, but all are associated with an abnormal haemoglobin. The sickle cell trait is found in nine per cent of American negroes, in parts of India and in 45 per cent of some African tribes. It is a chronic debilitating disease with symptoms of anaemia, thromboses in various organs or limbs and consequent pain and fever. There may be haemolytic or aplastic crises, often precipitated by infections. No coloured child should be treated for iron deficiency anaemia without sickle cell anaemia being considered. If there is no response to iron in four weeks, full laboratory investigation for sickling and other conditions should be carried out.

Thalassaemia (Cooley's anaemia) is a related condition with abnormally shaped red cells, occurring in the Mediterranean area or in those originating from that region. It is found in parts of India, Pakistan and Ceylon. In mild forms there is a mild persistent anaemia; in severe forms there is progressive severe anaemia with gross splenomegaly unless repeated transfusions are given. A characteristic facies develops owing to the thickening of the bones of the face and skull. The diagnosis is established by x-ray of bones, the reticulocytosis, the blood film, and haemoglobin electrophoresis. Thalassaemia may be associated with the sickle cell trait.

Glucose 6 phosphate dehydrogenase deficiency occurs in some millions of persons including Greeks, Cypriots, Turks, Chinese, Indians, Saudi Arabians, Filipinos and jews from Iran and Iraq. It leads to haemolysis particularly when certain drugs are administered, notably antimalarial drugs, B.A.L., diphenhydramine, naphthalene, nitrofurantoin, phenacetin, salicyclates sulphonamides and Vitamin K. Haemolysis may also occur if broad beans are eaten, and favism is due to the deficiency of this enzyme. Haemolysis may occur when certain infections occur, such as infective hepatitis or glandular fever. The diagnosis is made by enzyme assay, glutathione stability and the presence of Heinz bodies in the blood film. *Pyruvate kinase deficiency* is a rare enzyme deficiency associated with haemolysis.

Autoimmune haemolytic anaemia. This occurs in association with a variety of unrelated conditions, including virus infections (herpes, infective hepatitis), pyelonephritis, disseminated lupus erythematosus, periarteriis nodosa and dermatomyositis. The Coombs' test is positive. The diagnosis depends on laboratory investigations.

Drugs may cause haemolysis, apart from glucose 6 phosphate dehydrogenase deficiency. They include antimalarials, cephaloridine, chloramphenicol, cyclophosphamide, mefenamic acid, nalidixic acid, nitrofurantoin, P.A.S., penicillin, phenacetin, quinine, sulphonamides, troxidone and Vitamin K.

The haemolytic uraemic syndrome is a mysterious condition in which the child develops haemolytic anaemia, fever, abdominal pain, jaundice and signs of renal failure, often with thrombocytopenic purpura. There is commonly a mild gastroenteritis or upper respiratory tract infection, followed in two to five days by acute symptoms—vomiting, abdominal pain, oliguria or anuria, oedema, convulsions and intestinal haemorrhages. There may be hepatosplenomegaly. In the urine there are red cells, casts and albumin. Outbreaks have occurred in certain areas, but no infective or toxic

cause has been found. The diagnosis depends on the demonstration
of haemolysis, thrombocytopenia and renal failure, with characteristic burr cells (odd-shaped cells) in the blood smear. The condition
is more common in the first four years, especially the first year.
The mortality is high (about 40 per cent). Recovery follows in others
after four to eight weeks. The condition may be the same as throm-
botic thrombocytopenic purpura. Disseminated intravascular coagu-
lation may be the cause.

Nutritional anaemia

Prolonged breast feeding
Poor diet; mental deficiency
Anaemia of prematurity
Rickets
Scurvy
Steatorrhoea

By far the commonest cause of anaemia in a child after about
nine months of age is *nutritional anaemia.* This may be due to a
poor diet with inadequate protein and iron content, and an excess
of milk and carbohydrate. It occurs in tropical countries as a result
of prolonged breast feeding. One must not be deterred by a mother's
claim that the child is receiving a good mixed diet; such a history
is frequent, but there is no doubt that the child has not been receiving an appropriate diet. Mentally defective children (including
those with cerebral palsy) are liable to develop anaemia because of
the difficulty which many experience in chewing and therefore in
taking solid foods. They have to be maintained on thickened feeds,
and nutritional anaemia or avitaminoses are apt to develop.

The anaemia of prematurity is not strictly a nutritional anaemia,
but it is convenient to include it here. If small premature infants
are not given additional iron they are likely to become anaemic,
especially after the age of six months.

Nutritional rickets is itself associated with a hypochromic
anaemia. The diagnosis can be made in severe cases by the finding
of the markedly thickened epiphysis of the radius and ulna at the
wrist, but the diagnosis must be confirmed by x-ray of the wrist,

along with estimation of the plasma calcium, phosphorus and alkaline phosphatase.

Scurvy is now rarely seen, but is more likely to occur in defective children who are unable to chew and cannot take an ordinary mixed diet. The diagnosis is suggested by spongy bleeding gums, anaemia and severe pain in a leg due to subperiosteal haemorrhages.

The anaemia of *steatorrhoea* is due to the malabsorption, and so must be included under the heading of nutritional anaemia.

Defective red cell production

Infections
Drugs
Lead poisoning
Hypoplastic and aplastic anaemia
Megaloblastic anaemia
Thyroid deficiency
Miscellaneous
   Malignant disease
   Leukaemia
   Liver disease
   Bone disease
   Lipoid storage disease
   Letterer Siwe disease
   Uraemia

Infections. When a three or four week old baby gradually becomes anaemic, the cause may be a low-grade infection. The umbilicus must be examined for infection, and a blood culture should be performed if there is doubt. In the case of older infants and children, a low-grade infection, such as pyelonephritis, may cause a persistent mild anaemia.

Drugs. Numerous drugs are capable of causing anaemia. They include antiepileptic drugs, antihistamines, antimetabolites, azathiaprine, cephalexin, chloramphenicol, chlorothiazide, chlorpromazine, cycloserine, diazepoxide, gold, griseofulvin, imipramine, indomethacin, lincomycin, mefenamic acid, mepracine, meprobamate, methicillin, methimazole, P.A.S., phenacetin, phenothiazine, phenylbutazone, quinidine, ristocetin, salicylates, streptomycin, sulphonamides, tetracycline, thiobendazole, thiouracil and trimethoprim. Over 400 drugs or chemicals are known to cause blood dyscrasias. It follows that when a child presents with anaemia, one should ask in detail about all drugs taken in the previous few months. Various poisons, such as cleaning agents, paints, paint removers, lacquers and hydrocarbons may cause anaemia, often hypoplastic in type.

Lead poisoning in some areas, especially in low social classes, is an important cause of anaemia, especially where there is pica. It is commonly acquired by eating paint which is flaking off windowsills and other objects. Manifestations include abdominal pain, encephalopathy, headache, vomiting, anorexia, incoordination and weight loss. In severe cases there may be peripheral neuritis. Stippling of the red cells is unreliable. An x-ray may show increased density at the end of long bones, but the diagnosis is established by blood lead estimation.

Hypoplastic and aplastic anaemia may remain unexplained, after the fullest investigation, but it may be due to drugs and poisons, including lead, infections or exposure to irradiation. One form of hypoplastic anaemia (*Fanconi's* syndrome) is associated with skeletal deformities (notably an absent radius), skin pigmentation, hypogenitalism, dwarfism, microcephaly and webbed neck. In some cases there is an arrest in the maturation of the red cell for no discoverable reason, leading commonly to severe anaemia between the age of two and eighteen months. Many cases of 'hypoplastic' or 'aplastic' anaemia prove eventually to be due to leukaemia.

Megaloblastic anaemia may be due to steatorrhoea, pernicious anaemia, liver disease, drugs (anticonvulsants, nitrofurantoin), leukaemia and tapeworms. It may be caused by chronic infection in a malnourished child.

Cretinism may be associated with anaemia which responds to treatment with thyroxin.

A variety of other conditions cause anaemia, of which the most common is *malignant disease*, including leukaemia. Certain *bone diseases*, especially osteopetrosis, are associated with anaemia. *Renal failure* is usually accompanied by anaemia.

Conclusion

Anaemia in the newborn period is an acute emergency, requiring immediate hospital investigation and treatment.

Many children are treated with iron for a non-existent anaemia—and many other children, especially coloured ones, have an anaemia which is not diagnosed, and so do not receive treatment.

Iron deficiency is the commonest cause of anaemia after the newborn period, but the diagnosis should only be made with the help of a blood count. If there is not a good rise of the haemoglobin after treating a child with ferrous sulphate for a month, and if one can be sure that he really took the iron, the child should be properly investigated by a hospital laboratory.

For References—see p. 56.

Purpura

As the causes of purpura differ in the newborn baby from those in older children, the subject will be discussed in relation to the child's age.

The newborn

The main causes of purpura in the newborn baby are as follows:

Trauma
Maternal thrombocytopenia
Drug taken by the mother
Haemolytic disease
Septicaemia
Syphilis
Large naevus

Rare
  Congenital leukaemia

Toxoplasmosis
Cytomegalovirus
Galactosaemia
Rubella syndrome
Generalised herpes infection

Petechial haemorrhages over the face and forehead after birth
are normal. There may be obvious bruising as a result of delivery.
Petechiae occur particularly after severe anoxia. Retinal haemorrhages can be found in 19·2 per cent of all newborn babies, in 25·2
per cent of first-born babies, and in 52 per cent of those born by
vacuum extraction, but in none of those born by Caesarian section
(Schenker & Gombos, 1966).

When a mother has *thrombocytopenic purpura*, the baby may
have purpura for up to 12 weeks, with thrombocytopenia. This may
be due to a platelet agglutinin, or to an autoimmune process whereby maternal globulins have crossed into the foetus through the
placenta. Complete recovery is the rule (Scott, 1966).

Purpura in the infant may be the result of the mother taking
chlorothiazide or quinine in pregnancy.

Thrombocytopenia occurs in *haemolytic disease* due to rhesus or
ABO incompatibility.

When purpura develops in the newborn period, *septicaemia*
should be considered, especially if the baby is unwell.

When a baby has a *large cavernous haemangioma*, he may have
thrombocytopenic purpura. The mechanism is unknown, but it may
be due to adherence of the platelets to the haemangioma.

Congenital leukaemia, toxoplasmosis, cytomegalovirus infection
and *galactosaemia* are rare causes of purpura in the newborn.

Thrombocytopenic purpura in the newborn may be the result of
rubella during pregnancy.

The principal investigations necessary for diagnosis are a platelet
count, white cell count and film, investigation of the blood group,
blood culture for septicaemia, and if necessary serological tests for
rubella, toxoplasmosis and cytomegalovirus. A newborn baby with
purpura, other than petechial haemorrhages on the face and small
retinal haemorrhages, should be referred to a specialist for investigation.

Purpura after the newborn period

The common causes of purpura after the newborn period are as follows:

Trauma (e.g. child abuse)
Henoch Schönlein or anaphylactoid purpura
Idiopathic thrombocytopenic purpura
Leukaemia
The effect of drugs

Less common causes are:

Aplastic anaemia
Purpura with eczema (Aldrich's syndrome)
Disseminated lupus erythematosus
Haemolytic uraemic syndrome
Uraemia
Meningococcal septicaemia and other severe infections
Common infectious diseases
Haemophilia and allied diseases
Ehlers Danlos syndrome
Hereditary telangiectasia
Scurvy

Henoch Schönlein purpura is more common in boys than girls. It occurs particularly around the age of five or six years. Preceding haemolytic streptococcal infection is not usually a factor. There are commonly petechiae on the extensor surface of the limbs and around the buttocks, frequently associated with urticaria, effusion into joints and with abdominal pain and often bleeding from the bowel. The face is usually spared except in infants. Nephritis with haematuria complicates the condition in about 40 per cent of cases. Relapse is not uncommon. *Special investigations give entirely negative results*—an important diagnostic feature. The platelet count, bleeding and clotting time and capillary fragility tests are all normal. Provided that the diagnosis is correct, there is probably no indication for hospital treatment, as no specific treatment is available, but it would be unwise to keep at home an early case complicated by nephritis, because complications of nephritis (such as hypertensive encephalopathy) have to be treated in hospital. It would be a disaster to diagnose Henoch Schönlein purpura when the child in fact had meningococcal septicaemia.

Thrombocytopenic purpura is by far the commonest type of purpura in children after the Henoch Schönlein type. The child having been previously well is found to have bruises in various parts of the body without history of injury. It is more common between the age of three and seven than at other ages. The limbs are always involved, and there is commonly bleeding from the bowel, vagina or urinary tract. The course may be acute, lasting for three or four weeks, but it may last for many months. It is important to note that the spleen is not usually palpable; an enlarged spleen would strongly suggest some other diagnosis, such as leukaemia. The capillary fragility test is positive; the blood pressure cuff is inflated to a point halfway between the systolic and diastolic pressure, and is maintained for eight minutes. In a ring 2·5 cm in diameter 2·5 cm below the crease of the elbow the number of petechiae are counted half a minute after removal of the cuff. The test is positive if more than 20 are found. The diagnosis is confirmed in the laboratory by the prolonged bleeding time, thrombocytopenia and a normal blood film. It has to be distinguished above all from leukaemia by the blood film and bone marrow examination. A child with suspected thrombocytopenic purpura should be referred to a specialist for laboratory investigation, because other conditions may be confused with it and only eliminated by laboratory means. For instance, purpura may be due to meningococcal septicaemia, and a mistaken diagnosis would be likely to lead to the child's death.

The possibility that purpura may be due to *drugs* must always be remembered. Over 400 drugs or chemicals are known to cause blood dyscrasias. Those causing thrombocytopenia include such drugs as acetazolamide, actinomycin D, antiepileptic drugs, antihistamines, atropine, carbamazepine, cephalexin, chlordiazepoxide, chlorothiazide, chlorpheniramine, corticosteroids, iodides, meprobamate, methimazole, novobiocin, P.A.S., penicillin, phenylbutazone, phenytoin, quinidine, quinine, rifampicin, salicylates, sedormid, sulphadimidine, tolbutamide and trimethoprim. Numerous *poisons* affected the blood; they include paints, lacquers, paint removers and cleaning agents.

Purpura may be due to *hypoplastic* or *aplastic anaemia, Aldrich's syndrome* of eczema, purpura and recurrent infections, *disseminated lupus erythematosus* and the *haemolytic uraemic syndrome* (p. 48).

The possibility of *uraemia* should be remembered in an ill child with unexplained purpura at any age, including infancy. The blood pressure will be raised, and this part of the examination should not be forgotten.

Petechiae or ecchymoses are commonly found in *meningococcal septicaemia* (p. 31).

Purpura may occur in combination with *rubella, measles, chickenpox, scarlet fever, diphtheria* or *smallpox*. Purpura may follow *rubella* one to ten days after the onset of the rash.

A few petechiae may result from *whooping cough* or follow a *major convulsion*.

Bruising may be a feature of *haemophilia, Christmas disease*, and other bleeding disorders. A full laboratory investigation is essential. In *Von Willebrand's disease* there are epistaxes and bleeding from the gums and gastrointestinal tract. The bleeding time is prolonged, but the clotting time and platelet count are normal. The diagnosis is made by capillary microscopy and other means.

Purpura occurs in *hereditary telangiectasia*, in which telangiectases can be seen on the face, on the fingers and in the nasal or buccal mucosa, and in the *Ehlers-Danlos syndrome* in which there are over-extensible joints and a hyperelastic skin.

References

BALDINI M. (1966) Idiopathic thrombocytopenic purpura. *New Eng. J. Med.,* 274, 1245, 1301, 1360.

BAUM J.D. & BULPITT C.J. (1970) Retinal and conjunctival haemorrhage in the newborn. *Arch Dis. Childh.,* 45, 344.

HUGULEY C.M. (1966) Hematological reactions (Drugs). *J. Am. Med. Ass.,* 196, 408.

NADER P.R. & MARGOLIN F. (1966) Hemangioma causing gastrointestinal bleeding. *Am. J. Dis. Child.,* 111, 215.

NELIGAN G.A. & SMITH M.C. (1963) Prevention of haemorrhage from the umbilical cord. *Arch. Dis. Childh.,* 38, 471.

O'BRIEN R.T. & PEARSON H.A. (1971) Physiologic anaemias of the newborn infant, *J. Pediat.,* 79, 132.

PIEL C.F. & PHIBBS R.H. (1966) The hemolytic uremic syndrome. *Pediatric Clinics. N. America,* 13, 295.

Rausen A.R., Seki M. & Strauss L. (1965) Twin transfusion syndrome. *J. Pediat.*, 66, 613.

Scott J.S. (1966) Immunological diseases and pregnancy. *Brit. med. J.*, 1, 1559.

Poor appetite

I have discussed the problem of the poor appetite in detail elsewhere (Illingworth 1972). By far the commonest cause of a poor appetite, other than that due to an acute infection, is *food forcing*. This consists of feeding the child with a spoon, often by force, persuading him to eat more, offering him bribes if he will finish his dinner, threatening punishment if he does not eat, smacking him for not eating, allowing him to choose exactly what he would like to eat, allowing him to eat snacks at any time he likes between meals, and using various methods of distraction, so that when his attention is distracted some food can be put in by spoon.

Food forcing is itself due to a variety of causes, the chief of which are probably the following:

Excessive anxiety about the child's nutrition and weight

Dawdling with food—the child giving the impression that he has no appetite

The mother is apt to be concerned about the child's nutrition or weight because he is of *small build*.

She is apt to confuse the average weight with the normal weight—thinking that if the child is below the average weight, he must have something wrong with him. She does not realise that all children are different and that a child may be pounds below the average weight and yet be perfectly normal. Many mothers are concerned because the child's appetite is less in the second six months of his life than in the first six months. Mothers should be told how the weight gain falls off as the child grows older—averaging about

71 g per week from nine to 12 months, as compared with 170 o
198 g a week in the first three months—and the food intake is rela
tively less.

When babies are beginning to feed themselves, from nine to
about 18 months, they characteristically dawdle with their food
playing with it, patting it with the back of the spoon, and giving
the impression that they are not hungry. The mother then become
worried and tries to make them eat.

Well children vary in their appetite. There are little eaters and
big eaters. In general the active wiry child eats less than the
fat placid one. Efforts to make little eaters eat more always lead to
the opposite of the effect desired.

The mother's anxiety about her child's appetite is bound up with
many other factors. The problem is more common in an only
child or in a child born many years after the previous one. It is
more common when the parents are elderly and cannot have another child.

When food forcing occurs, food refusal results from two main
reasons. The child resists because of his normal negativism which
is a feature of the child aged about nine months to three years. In
addition the child becomes conditioned against food because whenever food is presented to him it is associated with unpleasantness,
forcing methods and often punishment, so that he develops a real
dislike for food.

Certain drugs may reduce the appetite—apart from amphetamine and the appetite suppressants. They include aminophylline,
amitriptlyline, antimetabolites, chlordiazepoxide, ephedrine, ethionamide, ethosuccimide, indomethacin, phenytoin, sulphasalazine and
Vitamin A or D excess.

If in addition to a poor appetite, the child does not appear well,
one must look for organic causes, such as chronic urinary tract infection, coeliac disease or other cause of 'failure to thrive' (p. 1).

Reference

ILLINGWORTH R.S. (1972) *The Normal Child*. 5th Edition. London, Churchill
    Livingstone.

Pica (dirt eating)

Pica, or dirt eating, occurs particularly in the first four or five years. It is more prevalent in the lower social classes than in the upper ones. It is more common in mentally defective children than in those of normal intelligence, partly because mentally defective children continue to take objects to the mouth long after the normal child has ceased to do so.

It has been thought by some that pica was associated with iron deficiency anaemia, but the association is often coincidental—iron deficiency anaemia and pica both being related to the low social class and to malnutrition. There is commonly a family history of pica, so that the child may have merely followed the example of others.

The danger of pica is the risk of infection, ingestion of worms and lead poisoning. In all cases the haemoglobin and blood lead should be determined.

References

CROSBY W.H. (1971) Food, pica and iron deficiency, *Arch. Int. Med.*, **127**, 960.

GUTELIUS M.F., MILLIGAN F.K., LAYMAN E.M., COHEN G.J. & DUBLIN C.C. (1962) Nutritional studies of children with pica. *Pediatrics*, **29**, 1012.

LOURIE R.S. (1965) *Clinical Proceedings, Children's Hospital of Columbia*, **21**, 193.

Nausea

Apart from the nausea which usually precedes vomiting, nausea is not a common symptom of childhood. The usual causes are:

Psychogenic, including distaste for school and attention seeking.
    Unpleasant sights or smells
Morning nausea
Dislike of certain foods

Vasomotor disturbance—posture, anaemia
Infective hepatitis
Fatty foods
Urinary tract infection
Cerebral tumour
Drugs

Nausea in the morning when *getting ready for school* may or may not represent the child's preference for staying at home. It is not always easy to be sure, because some children and adults do feel nausea in the morning—and have little breakfast. One needs to ask whether the morning nausea is as frequent in the weekends and holidays as it is in term time. Nausea may represent an attention-seeking device—when a mother expresses anxiety over the child's various symptoms.

Nausea on *changing posture* occurs in some older children. It is a vasomotor disturbance and is more common when there is anaemia.

Subclinical infective hepatitis may cause nausea and lassitude. Liver function tests, such as the serum glutamic oxalo-acetic transaminase (sgot) and the alkaline phosphatase, will help if the urine examination for bile does not reveal the diagnosis.

Urinary tract infection may show itself by vague unwellness and nausea.

It is a mistake to assume that the vomiting due to a *cerebral tumour* is not accompanied by nausea.

Numerous *drugs* may cause a feeling of nausea. They include amitriptyline, cephaloridine, chlordiazepoxide, diazepam, phenytoin, primidone, sulphasalazine and many others.

To establish the diagnosis a full physical examination is necessary, including culture of the urine in order to eliminate a urinary tract infection. Liver function tests will be carried out in a few cases.

Vomiting

It is probable that all children vomit, at least sometimes: but some vomit much more readily than others. Almost all normal babies bring some milk up after feeds. Either it wells up into the mouth, or else vomited material shoots out with a belch of wind. The difficulty lies in deciding whether vomiting can be disregarded as being within the range of normality, or whether investigation for disease is necessary.

The causes of vomiting are legion, and it would not be profitable to attempt to give a complete list of possible causes. Hence the discussion to follow is inevitably and intentionally incomplete; but I have tried to include the most important causes to consider when one is responsible for assessing a vomiting child. For convenience I have related the discussion to three age periods—the newborn infant, the infant after the newborn period, and the child after infancy. There will be some overlapping between these three groupings.

The newborn infant

The following causes of vomiting may be important:

Normal possetting
Sucking and swallowing difficulties
Possible gastric irritation
Oesophageal atresia or stenosis
Perforation of the pharynx
Chalasia of the oesophagus
Vascular ring
Duodenal stenosis
Meconium plug or ileus
Intestinal atresia
Lactobezoar
Hirschsprung's disease (p. 14)
Drugs and poisons

61

Infections, including meningitis, septicaemia
Cerebral causes, including subdural effusion
Kernicterus
Metabolic disorders—phenylketonuria, galactosaemia, carbohydrate
    intolerance, hypervalinaemia, adrenocortical hyperplasia
Renal causes—urethral obstruction, renal insufficiency

It is common for the normal newborn baby to bring some milk up after feeds. When the vomiting is frequent one has to consider the possibility of organic disease. When only small amounts come up after feeds and the child is well, taking the feeds normally and gaining weight (after the first two or three days), it is likely that no disease is responsible. It has been suggested, on what evidence I am not sure, that much vomiting in the newborn period is due to irritation of the stomach by amniotic contents, meconium or blood swallowed during delivery. Since all babies in utero constantly swallow amniotic fluid, it seems unlikely that amniotic fluid would cause vomiting after birth. It is at least true to say that some newborn babies vomit fairly frequently in the first few days after birth, sometimes causing anxiety, and then settle down without further trouble and without treatment.

The features which would make one seriously consider organic disease are as follows:

(1) Persistent vomiting, as distinct from occasional vomiting.

(2) The presence of bile in the vomit (green vomitus). This would suggest obstruction below the ampulla of Vater, but green vomitus may occur when there is a serious infection or birth injury. *Green vomitus should be regarded as being due to intestinal obstruction until proved otherwise.* Green vomitus should be distinguished from yellow colostrum or from vomitus containing meconium.

(3) Drowsiness, failure to suck well, failure to demand feeds.

(4) Abdominal distension. This suggests obstruction in the lower part of the intestinal tract. There is commonly no distension in the presence of high intestinal obstruction.

(5) Failure to gain weight or loss of weight.

(6) Dehydration.

(7) Fever. This may be due to dehydration or infection.

(8) Failure to pass meconium in the first 24 hours. This suggests

meconium ileus, Hirschsprung's disease or intestinal obstruction. The passage of a stool in the first 24 hours does not, however, exclude obstruction.

(9) Visible peristalsis from right to left, suggesting obstruction in the jejunum, ileum or colon.

(10) The presence of a palpable mass—meconium ileus, enlarged kidneys, reduplication of the intestine or a palpable bladder.

(11) The presence of a bulging fontanelle, suggesting cerebral oedema or an intracranial haemorrhage.

These and other conditions will now be discussed in more detail.

Obstruction in the alimentary tract

Hirschsprung's disease is perhaps the commonest cause of intestinal obstruction in the newborn (see p. 14).

Atresia of the oesophagus is suggested when the infant's mother had hydramnios. In such a case it is the practice to pass a catheter down the infant's oesophagus immediately after birth, in order to make sure that there is no atresia and until that has been done a feed must not be given. If there is atresia, the catheter commonly meets an obstruction four inches (10 cm) from the lips. The lower end of the catheter may coil itself in the blind upper pouch of the oesophagus, and one may be misled unless an x-ray photograph is taken. Atresia is suspected when the infant's mouth is overflowing with mucus and saliva. It will be suspected when a baby chokes and vomits on being given his first feed, or vomits nothing but mucus between feeds. The diagnosis of atresia is usually confirmed by a straight x-ray (without lipiodol).

According to Ducharme *et al.* (1971) *perforation of the pharynx* in the new-born causes symptoms identical with those of oesophageal atresia. It may be impossible to pass a nasogastric tube in both conditions, and radiological studies are confusing. A *vascular ring* will be considered if there is stridor, usually inspiratory and expiratory, commonly with vomiting. *Chalasia of the oesophagus*, or lax cardio-oesophageal sphincter, is an unusual cause of vomiting in the new-born period. Theoretically the vomiting should only occur when the child is lying down, but in practice this is unreliable.

Duodenal stenosis would be suspected when a baby vomits repeatedly without abdominal distension. Bile will be present in the vomitus only when the obstruction is below the ampulla. Duodenal stenosis of atresia may be a feature in mongols.

A *meconium plug* consists of greyish brown inspissated material which precedes the passage of normal meconium. The plug may sometimes be expelled after digital examination of the rectum.

Meconium ileus may be suspected when meconium is not passed in the first 24 hours. Multiple masses may sometimes be felt in the distended abdomen. As it is usually a manifestation of fibrocystic disease of the pancreas, there may be a history of that condition in a sibling.

Intestinal atresia may be associated with other congenital abnormalities of the alimentary tract, such as oesophageal atresia or imperforate anus. The symptoms and signs are persistent vomiting with bile in the vomitus, abdominal distension, often visible peristalsis and constipation. Vomiting tends to occur later and to be less profuse when the obstruction is in the lower part of the alimentary tract, but distension is more marked. Obstruction may be caused by malrotation or volvulus. Vomiting, blood in the stool and abdominal distension may follow perforation of the colon after a replacement transfusion (p. 114). Obstruction a few days after birth may result from inspissated milk (lactobezoar), usually resulting from milk being insufficiently diluted (Cook and Rickham 1969).

If there is one anomaly of the alimentary tract, such as an imperforate anus, there is a risk that there is another anomaly, such as a tracheo-oesophageal fistula or duodenal stenosis.

Ganglion-blocking drugs given in pregnancy to the mother for hypertension may be followed by ileus in the newborn baby for the first week or two.

Infection

A second serious cause of vomiting in the newborn period is an infection. This may be septicaemia, resulting from an infected umbilicus. Other infections include meningitis and gastroenteritis. *Meningitis in the young baby is commonly manifested by drowsiness, loss of appetite, vomiting and sometimes by fits. There may or may not be a bulging fontanelle. There is commonly no neck stiffness or other sign of meningism. The unexplained drowsiness and illness without other discoverable cause leads one to carry out a lumbar puncture in order to exclude pyogenic meningitis. The diagnosis of this condition is a matter of great urgency. Delay in instituting treatment is likely to be fatal or to lead to serious permanent sequelae, such as mental deficiency.*

In a serious infection the vomited material may be green, as in the case of intestinal obstruction.

Cerebral damage or defect

Vomiting may be an important symptom of *cerebral oedema* or of an *intracranial haemorrhage*, such as a *subdural haematoma*. The signs are often bulging of the fontanelle and wide separation of the sutures. The child may have an abnormal high-pitched cry and be unduly drowsy or irritable—showing an exaggerated startle reflex and even twitching, frank convulsions or cyanotic attacks. The Moro reflex may be exaggerated or absent. Ophthalmoscopic examination may show retinal haemorrhages—though it must be remembered that small haemorrhages may be found in normal newborn babies. Vomited material may be green. Depression of the respiratory centre as a result of the increased intracranial pressure may cause atelectasis, so that respiratory symptoms may outweigh the cerebral ones.

The diagnosis of a *subdural haematoma* must be made by subdural taps. Failure to diagnose a subdural haematoma causes serious brain damage and progressive hydrocephalus.

Kernicterus should no longer be seen now, because it can be prevented by replacement transfusion when the serum bilirubin reaches a dangerous level. Symptoms usually commence about the fifth to the ninth day, and consist of vomiting, loss of appetite, arching of the back, spasticity, rolling of the eyes and sometimes convulsions. There may be a peculiar pronation of the wrist.

Metabolic causes of vomiting include phenylketonuria, galactosaemia, lactose or fructose intolerance and adrenocortical hyperplasia. Vomiting due to these causes may occur in the newborn period, but is usually later. The diagnosis of *phenylketonuria* has to be suspected when a sibling has the disease; phenylpyruvic acid does not usually appear in the urine for the first four or five weeks, and the diagnosis should be made immediately after birth by estimation of the serum phenylalanine and tyrosine.

Another rare cause of vomiting in the young baby is *hypervalinaemia*.

Renal causes of vomiting include *hydronephrosis* from urethral obstruction. A useful pointer to the diagnosis would be a distended bladder with a poor urinary stream—or failure to pass urine.

For sucking and swallowing difficulties, see p. 135; for vascular ring, see p. 151.

Infancy after the newborn period

The following causes should be considered:

(1) Non-organic
   Normal possetting. Food coming up with wind
   Incorrect feeds
   Overfeeding (premature babies only)
   Careless handling after feeds
   Rumination
   Giving solids before the baby can chew
   Delay in giving solids
   Crying causing vomiting
   Travel sickness
   Migraine

(2) Organic
   Congenital pyloric stenosis
   Hiatus hernia, chalasia of the oesophagus
   Infection
   Whooping cough
   Winter vomiting disease
   Coeliac disease
   Other metabolic causes
      Phenylketonuria
      Galactosaemia

Carbohydrate intolerance
Ketotic hypoglycaemia
Adrenocorticol hyperplasia
Intussusception or other intestinal obstruction
Appendicitis
Diabetic acidosis
Uraemia
Increased intracranial pressure
Drugs or poisons

Probably all normal infants bring some milk up after feeds, but some bring up more than others, or bring it up more frequently. The difficulty in such cases lies in deciding whether the vomiting is within normal limits or not, and so whether it is desirable to investigate for organic disease.

The first feature which guides one is the weight gain. If there is a story of vomiting over a prolonged period, and the child's weight in relation to his birth weight is average or above average, one is less likely to miss organic disease than in an underweight infant. One is frequently asked to see an infant who is said to have vomited the whole of every feed every day for some weeks, and who is above the average weight for the age. One then knows that the mother, in her anxiety or desire to impress, is exaggerating. It would not be safe to assume that organic disease in such a child could be absolutely excluded, for he might have a hiatus hernia. Organic disease is more likely if the child is underweight.

Another feature of importance would be the presence of blood in the vomitus, for that would suggest *hiatus hernia* or *reflux* due to chalasia of the oesophagus.

By far the commonest non-organic cause of vomiting is *excessive wind*. In a breast fed baby this is due to the baby sucking too long on the breast, or sucking on an empty breast so that he swallows air. Sometimes a breast fed baby swallows air as a result of gulping milk rapidly. He does this not because he is 'greedy', but because the milk is flowing out of the breast rapidly—usually at the first feed in the morning, when the breast is distended. The young baby commonly does not bring his lips tightly round the nipple and sucks in air at the angle of the mouth. In a bottle fed baby the almost invariable cause of excessive wind is the presence of too small a hole in the teat. A bottle feed should not take more than ten or 15 minutes. I am repeatedly told by mothers of 'windy' babies that the feeds take 45 to 60 minutes. All that time the baby is swallowing air. A baby may also swallow an excess of air if he is allowed to suck when the teat has flattened as a result of a vacuum having been created in the bottle. For the same reason the baby may suffer from wind if he is left to suck on a bottle which has been propped up on a pillow. Two babies were referred to me on account of excessive wind because the mother in each case had filled the bottle with sago pudding and expected the baby to be able to suck it through the teat.

Theoretically the baby may be sick as a result of wrong food. In fact this is rare in my experience, though one must always ask a mother not just how much milk the baby is being given, but how much milk powder, sugar and water is being given at each feed. I have seen some impressive mistakes made by them. It is a regrettable fact that many doctors and nurses, when faced with a baby who cries, vomits, or has other symptoms, still advise mothers to change from one dried food to another in order to find one which 'suits' the baby. The differences between the dried milks are so trivial that *it is never necessary to change from one dried milk to another*, except in the case of the rare metabolic diseases such as hypercalcaemia or carbohydrate intolerance. Yet I have seen hundreds of babies who have been tried on one dried milk after another in an effort to find one which 'suits' the baby—when his symptoms were due to something different, such as congenital pyloric stenosis.

Some would say that *overfeeding* is an important cause of vomiting.

Careless handling of the baby after a feed may cause milk to be brought up. This applies particularly to the premature baby in which the cardiooesophageal sphincter is lax. If his nappy is changed after a feed, and the buttocks and therefore lower part of the body are elevated, milk may be brought up.

Rumination is an unusual non-organic cause of vomiting. The baby, aged usually six months to a year, but sometimes older, seems to try to get the milk up, pushes his abdomen in and out, arches his back, and eventually brings it up. He may make sucking movements with his lips or cheeks, and is apt to stop his action if watched. It is commonly ascribed to emotional deprivation, but it is wise to eliminate a hiatus hernia by radiological examination.

A baby is likely to vomit if *given solids before he can chew*. Most babies begin to chew at six or seven months; they can be given thickened feeds before then, but not solids. A retarded child is later than the normal child in beginning to chew, and so is liable to vomit from this cause. If a child is not given solids at a time when he has recently become able to chew, he is likely to refuse solids and to vomit them. This probably depends on the sensitive or critical period (Illingworth & Lister, 1964).

Some infants may develop a strong *dislike for certain foods*, and vomit them if the mother insists on giving these foods. Some mothers force their infants to take certain foods which are thought to be good for them, or try to compel them to take more than they need, with the result that they vomit.

Some infants have an unfortunate way of vomiting if they are *left to cry* for any length of time. This may be due to air swallowing when crying, or to putting his thumb or finger into the back of the throat.

Travel sickness may begin in young infants five or six months of age.

Migraine begins as a vomiting. It may first appear in infancy (p. 91).

Allergy to cow's milk is a rare cause of vomiting.

Vomiting is *not* due to teething.

An *organic cause* for vomiting would be suspected if the child suddenly began to vomit after being previously well; if he were ill or febrile in addition to vomiting; if there were other symptoms; if he had an inadequate weight gain or lost weight; or if there were blood in the vomitus.

Congenital pyloric stenosis occurs in one in 150 boys and one in 775 girls. There is a genetic factor. The onset of vomiting is nearly always between four and six weeks of age, though rarely it can begin in the newborn period. If vomiting begins after the age of ten weeks, it is exceedingly unlikely to be due to pyloric stenosis.

The essential feature is projectile vomiting immediately after or during a feed. There is one big vomit and almost the whole feed comes up. If the baby is merely bringing small quantities up at intervals between one feed and the next, e.g., an hour or two after a feed, pyloric stenosis can be almost excluded. Rarely a child may have one big vomit immediately after or during a feed, and bring small quantities up for an hour or two, like a normal baby frequently does; but this is an unusual picture. There is no bile in the vomitus. The vomiting begins with one feed and may then occur in every subsequent feed or not until the next day. It rapidly becomes more frequent, so that in two or three days the baby is vomiting at almost every feed. As a result of the vomiting the baby becomes constipated and dehydrated. Peristaltic waves may be seen crossing from left to right in the upper abdomen. The expert will feel a pyloric tumour which comes and goes and is commonly of the size of a pea, slightly to the right of the umbilicus and usually a little above. He feels the baby during a feed. If the stomach is distended when he is about to begin, he will wash the stomach out first, because it is often impossible to feel a tumour when the stomach is distended.

Owing to the infrequency with which pyloric stenosis is seen in general practice, the family doctor should not rely on his ability to feel the tumour. He should suspect the diagnosis and ask the paediatrician to express an opinion on examination. The diagnosis is established by feeling the tumour. X-ray examination is nearly always unnecessary. There is no place for a therapeutic test of atropine methyl nitrate, for the correct treatment is surgical. The majority of babies with congenital pyloric stenosis seen in hospital have been tried on one dried food after another to find one which suits the baby.

Pylorospasm in my opinion is probably a non-existent condition in infants, though some will disagree. I can certainly say that I have never recognised a case, or seen a case thought by someone else to be pylorospasm and which did not appear to me to be incorrectly diagnosed. I have seen no evidence that such a condition exists. I usually find that babies thought to have this condition are suffering from excessive wind, congenital pyloric stenosis or are merely normal 'possetters'.

Chalasia of the oesophagus and *hiatus hernia* should always be suspected in a vomiting baby if there is blood in the vomitus. If this is the case, a barium swallow x-ray should be performed. I would certainly have this done if a vomiting baby were also anaemic, because of the possibility of a hiatus hernia, or if there were much vomiting or loss of weight. One has also to be guided by the degree of the mother's anxiety. Sometimes a really anxious mother is not reassured until an x-ray examination has been performed. One has to balance this against the irradiation which a barium swallow involves.

When a previously well infant becomes ill and vomits, the possible causes are numerous. The most likely is an *infection*. These include otitis media, gastroenteritis, urinary tract infection, whooping cough, 'winter vomiting' and meningitis. Otitis media is suspected when an infant has a cold or has just recovered from one, and is readily diagnosed by the auriscope. Gastroenteritis may cause some difficulty in the diagnosis for a few hours, in that vomiting may precede diarrhoea. A history of diarrhoea in another member of the family makes the diagnosis easier. The possibility of a urinary tract infection must not be forgotten. *Ketotic hypoglycaemia* may present as vomiting and fits. This occurs particularly in children who were of low birthweight.

Whooping cough is an important cause of vomiting (p. 141).

The term *'winter vomiting'* disease is not a good one, for it occurs in summer and winter. It is almost certainly a virus infection, but attempts to isolate the virus have failed. It has been well described in a report by the College of Practitioners, in which 1300 cases were recorded by 106 family doctors. It is highly infectious, with an incubation period of one to three days. Haworth *et al.* (1956) found a pleocytosis in the cerebrospinal fluid of all three children in whom a lumbar puncture was carried out, and suggested that a neurotropic virus might be responsible. Normally the only symptom is vomiting, nearly always in the night. Diarrhoea, if it occurs at all, is most unusual. The child is afebrile and is well until he suddenly vomits without previous nausea and without warning. The vomiting may recur.

Drugs and Poisons. Innumerable drugs may cause vomiting. Poisoning should always be considered when a previously well child begins to vomit without discoverable cause. It must always be remembered that the possibility of poisoning may be stoutly denied by a parent—either because the parent genuinely does not know that the child has ingested drugs or other poison, or because he does not want to admit that the child has access to them. One of my colleagues described five cases of salicylate poisoning in which the diagnosis was made difficult by sustained denial by the parents that the children could possibly have had access to the drugs (Pickering, 1964).

Vomiting after infancy

Non-organic causes

Vomiting because of psychological factors is common in children. These causes may be grouped as follows:

(1) Excitement. Some children may vomit as the result of excitement, such as the prospect of going to a party.

(2) Fear or anxiety. Anxiety about going to school, or about leaving home, may cause vomiting in school-age children in the morning before departure for school.

(3) Suggestion and imitation. Vomiting may be suggested by anxious parents on a car journey. Vomiting may result from the child seeing another child vomit.

(4) Attention-seeking device. Vomiting may occur as an attention-seeking device if the child sees that sickness causes consternation and anxiety.

(5) Insertion of finger into throat. Some small children make themselves sick, probably accidentally, by insertion of a finger into the throat—sometimes when the throat is sore as a result of tonsillitis.

(6) Migraine. Though it may be argued that migraine is an example of organic disease, emotional factors may precipitate attacks. Migraine, also termed in children the periodic syndrome, is described elsewhere.

(7) Travel sickness.

Organic causes are suggested if the vomiting is of sudden onset, or if the child in between attacks of vomiting is not well and is lacking in energy—though these symptoms may be psychological in origin. They are certainly suggested if there is loss of weight. It must not be forgotten that the periodic syndrome can be confused with other conditions such as recurrent volvulus, herniation of the stomach through the diaphragm, ketotic hypoglycaemia, or recurrent urinary tract infection; and that even if a child is known to suffer from migraine, he may also develop a different condition such as acute appendicitis, which also causes abdominal pain and vomiting.

Organic causes include the following:

Infection, especially tonsillitis or otitis media
  Meningitis
  Winter vomiting disease
Appendicitis, mesenteric lymphadenitis
Intestinal obstruction
Torsion of the testis (p. 107)
Poisons and drugs

As in the younger child, the commonest organic cause of vomiting is *an infection*—such as otitis media, tonsillitis, pyelonephritis, whooping cough, gastroenteritis or the winter vomiting disease. Meningitis is another possible cause, but in the case of the older child signs of meningism are usually but not invariably present.

Unexplained vomiting may be due to *drugs* or *poisons*. Innumerable medicines cause vomiting. They include anthelmintics, antibiotics, antidepressants, antiepileptic drugs, antihistamines, antimitotic drugs, morphia, pethidine, salicylates, tranquillisers, drugs given for rheumatic fever and other drugs.

Vomiting may be a symptom of *lead poisoning*.

References

College of Practitioners (No date) Epidemic winter vomiting. Symposium by the Epidemic Observation Unit of the College of General Practitioners. *Research News Letter No. 8.*

Cook R.C.M., Rickham P.P. (1969) Neonatal intestinal obstruction due to milk curds. *J. Pediat. Surgery*, 4, 599.

Ducharme J.C., Bertrand R. & Debie J. (1971) Perforation of the pharynx in the newborn. A condition mimicking oesophageal atresia. *Can. Med. Ass. J.*, 104, 785.

FRASER G.C. & WILKINSON A.W. (1967) Neonatal Hirschsprung's Disease. *Br. med. J.*, **2**, 7.

HAWORTH J.C., TYRELL D.A.J. & WHITEHEAD J.E.M. (1956) Winter vomiting disease with meningeal involvement. *Lancet*, **2**, 1152.

ILLINGWORTH R.S. & LISTER J. (1964) The critical or sensitive period, with special reference to certain feeding problems in infants and children. *J. Pediat.*, **65**, 839.

JONES P.G. (1970) *Clinical Paediatric Surgery*. Bristol, John Wright.

MENKING M., WAGNITZ J.G., BURTON J.J., CODDINGTON R.D. and SOTOS J.F. (1969) Rumination, a near fatal psychiatric disease of infancy. *New Engl. J. Med.*, **280**, 802.

PICKERING D. (1964) Salicylate poisoning: The diagnosis when its possibility is denied by the parents. *Acta Paediat. Uppsala*, **53**, 501.

Haematemesis

When a child brings blood up from the stomach, the following are the conditions to consider first:

In a newborn infant
  Swallowed blood during delivery
  Swallowed blood from the mother's nipple
  Haemorrhagic disease of the newborn

Infancy after the newborn period
  Hiatus hernia
  Chalasia of the oesophagus
  Blood diseases

After infancy
  Hiatus hernia
  Severe retching for any reason
  Nose bleeds
  Acute tonsillitis
  Oesophageal varices
  Aspirin or other salicylates
  Peptic ulcer (e.g. during corticosteroid treatment)

Zollinger–Ellison syndrome (rare)
Intestinal obstruction (altered blood)
Blood diseases
Uraemia
Poisons (e.g. corrosive substances, ferrous sulphate)

When a newborn baby in his first three or four days vomits blood, one needs to know whether it is the baby's blood or the mother's blood. He may have swallowed the mother's blood during delivery, or have swallowed blood from the mother's cracked nipple. The two are readily distinguished by the chemical test described on p. 45. If it is the baby's blood, the most likely cause is haemorrhagic disease of the newborn, commonly due to hypoprothrombinaemia. In this case he requires treatment, and a careful watch must be kept to ensure that the blood loss is not such that a transfusion is necessary.

After the newborn period, when a baby brings up streaks of blood in the vomitus, the commonest causes are *hiatus hernia* or *chalasia*. It is rare in pyloric stenosis.

At any age haematemesis may be a feature of *blood diseases*.

Severe retching for any reason may lead to streaking of vomitus with blood.

Other causes of blood in the vomitus of a child are *blood swallowed after a nose bleed or from acute tonsillitis*—presumably as a result of rupture of a blood vessel in the acutely inflamed throat.

Oesophageal varices only occur in association with *cirrhosis of the liver, portal hypertension or hypersplenism*.

Polycystic disease of the liver and kidney is an unusual cause of haematemesis.

Aspirin may cause bleeding from the stomach. Salicylates in an overdosage may cause bleeding by hypoprothrombinaemia or thrombocytopenia. Haematemesis may result from an overdose of animophyllin. The possibility of *poisoning* by a corrosive substance or other material (such as ferrous sulphate), or boric acid poisoning, must never be forgotten.

Peptic ulceration may occur in children, though it is a rare cause of haematemesis. The possibility should be remembered when a child receiving corticosteriods complains of abdominal pain.

The Zollinger–Ellison syndrome is more common in boys; it consists of peptic ulceration with a non-beta cell islet tumour of the pancreas. The symptoms include abdominal pain, vomiting, haematemesis, diarrhoea and melaena.

Finally, altered blood in the vomitus is a feature of *intestinal obstruction*.

Constipation

The following conditions should be considered:

Newborn
   Obstruction of the alimentary tract
   Hirschsprung's disease (p. 14)
   Meconium plug
Later infancy and childhood
   Breast fed
     excess of protein or fat in the mother's diet
   Artificially fed
     undiluted cow's milk
     insufficient milk, sugar or water
     result of vomiting
     normal variation
   Mismanagement of toilet training
   Hirschsprung's disease
   Result of laxatives or other drugs
   Rare
     anorectal stenosis
     cretinism
     hypotonia
     lead poisoning
     metabolic conditions associated with polyuria

Distinguish the infrequent stools of a fully breast-fed baby.

Ninety per cent of infants pass meconium in the first 24 hours. Delay in passing meconium (e.g. until after 36 hours) strongly suggests an obstruction in the alimentary tract or Hirschsprung's disease. The delay may be due to nothing more than a meconium plug which may be released by a finger on rectal examination. Constipation in the newborn baby may be due to immaturity of the nervous mechanism.

The fully breast-fed infant may have infrequent stools, but this is not constipation. It is common for a fully breast-fed infant to have only one stool every four or five days. I have seen two infants who regularly had one stool every 12 days, and they were entirely normal. The stools are soft and semi-liquid, as those of a breast-fed baby who has a stool every day or two. Infrequent stools are perfectly normal and no treatment is required. If a breast-fed infant has Hirschsprung's disease, the stools may be hard. If the mother of a fully breast-fed baby takes a considerable excess of fat or protein, the infant's stools may be bulky and offensive and unduly firm, but not usually loose.

A common cause of constipation in an artificially fed baby is *deficiency of fluid in the feed, insufficiency of milk or insufficiency of sugar*. In hot weather or in a hot climate the infant must have more than the customary 148 ml of fluid per kg per day. If a child is overclothed and so perspires excessively, he will lose fluid and may be constipated. Constipation occurs in some infants if undiluted cow's milk is given.

Anything which causes vomiting, such as *excessive possetting* or *pyloric stenosis*, will cause constipation.

It is not known why some artificially fed babies become constipated on a diet on which other infants have normal stools. There are evidently differences in the amount of fluid absorption in the intestine and differences in the pattern of peristalsis. It is known that more water is absorbed from the stools in the rectum of constipated children than from others, and there is greater muscle tone in the terminal colon. It is probable that there are genetic and constitutional factors which affect the consistency of the stools, apart altogether from the nature of the food given, and the quantity of fluid taken. It is almost certainly incorrect to ascribe all constipation in young children to psychological causes. In a study of 210 constipated children (Davidson, 1963), 61 per cent had been constipated before the age of six months, 50 per cent had parents with functional gastrointestinal symptoms, and 40 per cent had siblings with similar symptoms. Nevertheless, psychological factors may add to the problem. When a mother expresses anxiety about the child's toilet training and bowel movements, the child is likely to sense the anxiety and respond by withholding stools. This will almost certainly be the case if the mother compels him to sit on the pottie when he is trying to get off it, or if she smacks him for not passing a stool. Punishment inhibits the defaecation reflex. The constipation is likely to begin as a result of dietary, genetic and constitutional factors, and to continue and to be aggravated by mismanagement. Faulty and excessive bowel training is probably the principal cause of constipation. If a child finds it painful to pass a stool because it is hard or because he has an anal fissure, he may as a result withhold stools and become constipated.

There is no need for a child to have a stool every day. Mothers have a greatly exaggerated idea of the significance of constipation. Provided that when the stool comes it is not hard, it does not matter if there is an interval of two or three days between stools.

The use of *laxatives*, which are rarely necessary in infants and young children, may itself lead to constipation. There is insufficient bulk in the remaining stool to stimulate peristalsis and so defaecation. *Various drugs* may cause constipation. They include chlordiazepoxide, amitriptyline, imipramine and vincristine.

A rare cause of constipation is *anorectal stenosis*. The stool may resemble the passage of toothpaste from a tube. A rectal examination will establish the diagnosis.

Rare causes of constipation include *cretinism*, *hypotonia*, and *lead poisoning*.

Certain *metabolic conditions* which are associated with polyuria may lead to constipation. They include diabetes insipidus, hypercalcaemia, renal acidosis, and the salt-losing type of adrenocortical hyperplasia. If on examining a child suffering from the 'failure to thrive' syndrome, one found numerous faecal masses in the abdomen, one would strongly suspect one of the above conditions.

References

DAVIDSON M. (1963) Natural history of chronic constipation. *Forty-fourth Ross Conference on Pediatric Research*, p. 65.

DAVIDSON M., KUGLER M.M. & BAUER C.H. (1963) Diagnosis and management in children with severe and protracted constipation and obstipation. *J. Pediat.*, **62,** 261.

ELLIS D. & CLATWORTHY H.W. (1966) The meconium plug syndrome revisited. *J. Pediat. Surgery*, **1,** 54.

FRASER G.C., WILKINSON A.W. (1967) Neonatal Hirschsprung's Disease. *Brit. Med. J.*, **2,** 7.

ROSENBLUD M.L. (1967) Zollinger–Ellison syndrome in children. *Am. J. med. Sci.*, **254,** 884.

WOODMANSEY A.C. (1967) Emotion and the motions. *Br. J. Med. Psychol.*, **40,** 207.

Diarrhoea

Many infants and children are said by their mothers to have diarrhoea when in fact their stools are normal.

Fully breast-fed babies always have loose stools, unless they have Hirschsprung's disease. Their stools are explosive, contain curds (in the early weeks), and may be bright green in colour. They may be frequent, as many as 24 stools in the 24 hours. Fully breast-fed babies virtually never suffer from gastroenteritis.

The so-called *starvation stools* may be confused with diarrhoea. These are loose green frequent small stools, containing little faecal matter. They are due to gross deficiency of food intake. It is a disaster if further restriction of food occurs on the grounds that the child has gastroenteritis or is being overfed. *Overfeeding* does not cause diarrhoea. Many infants are said to be suffering from overfeeding when the correct diagnosis is underfeeding.

Many older children are referred to the paediatrician on account of chronic diarrhoea and on examination it is found that they are up to the average in weight. If the mother is asked to bring sample stools on a subsequent occasion, it is found that they are entirely normal. It is always important to see the stools if there are reasons for doubting the mother's story.

It is vital to remember that *diarrhoea is never due to teething*.

When a baby presents with true diarrhoea, the following conditions should be considered:

Too much sugar in the feed
Gastroenteritis
Necrotising enterocolitis
Diarrhoea in association with parenteral infection
Hirschsprung's disease (p. 14)
Carbohydrate intolerance and malabsorption (p. 12)
Steatorrhoea (p. 10)
Protein-losing enteropathy (p. 13)
Drugs and poisons

In older children causes include:

   Emotional stress
   Constipation—pseudodiarrhoea
   Allergy
   Irritable colon syndrome
Rare
   Chronic infections of the alimentary tract
   Ulcerative colitis
   Regional ileitis and Crohn's disease of the colon
   Appendicitis, intussusception
   Ganglioneuroma
   Thyrotoxicosis
   Pancreatic insufficiency with neutropenia
   Zollinger–Ellison syndrome
   Adrenocortical hyperplasia

When artificially fed babies develop diarrhoea, the likely causes are *an excess of sugar in the feed* or *gastroenteritis*. Orange juice gives some babies looseness of the stools. When an artificially fed baby has mild chronic looseness of the stools, it is well to cut out the sugar altogether in order to determine whether it is the sugar which is the cause of the trouble.

Infective *gastroenteritis* is most commonly due to contamination of food, but may be due to a respiratory tract virus. It is surprising how many lay people ascribe diarrhoea on holiday in Spain to 'the heat', or to 'the cooking', when it is obvious that the diarrhoea is due to infection. An important cause of diarrhoea in young babies is *Hirschsprung's disease*. *Neonatal necrotising entercolitis* is a serious disease affecting mainly low birthweight babies, especially if they were anoxic at birth. The cause is unknown. The infant becomes poorly, brings up bile stained vomit and sometimes has diarrhoea.

Many infants develop diarrhoea following an *upper respiratory tract infection* such as a cold or otitis media. Some infants develop diarrhoea in association with a urinary tract infection (pyelonephritis).

Several *drugs* cause diarrhoea. They include in particular the antibiotics, such as penicillin by mouth or the tetracyclines. Iron medicine may occasionally cause diarrhoea in a child, but it is unusual. A child referred to me on account of diarrhoea was found to be receiving a laxative every night from the father without the knowledge of the child's mother. Other drugs sometimes causing diarrhoea include antimetabolites, bephenium, carbamazepine, cephalexin, dichlorophen, ethionamide, fenfluramine, flufenamic acid, griseofulvin, indomethacin, kanamycin, lincomycin, mefenamic acid, nalidixic acid, nystatin, P.A.S., paromomycin, phenothiazines, rifampicin, sodium fusidate, thiobendazole, thyroxin overdose, vancomycin and viprynium. It is possible that a fully breast fed baby may have diarrhoea because of a laxative (senna, cascara, rhubarb or aloes) taken by the mother.

Emotional stress in an older child may cause mild diarrhoea. Such stress may be due to fear of a particular teacher, fear of bullying or other anxieties.

The complaint that a child has soiling of his pants with diarrhoea usually signifies *constipation with overflow* (see encopresis). The diagnosis is made by rectal examination.

A rare cause of diarrhoea is *allergy*, and the most common form of this is milk protein allergy. I should be unwilling to accept this diagnosis unless there were a clear history that the diarrhoea only occurs when milk is given, and that if milk substitutes are given (such as soya bean preparations) there is no diarrhoea. There should be a recurrence on reintroducing milk. It would be essential to investigate for carbohydrate intolerance which is usually associated with diarrhoea.

The irritable colon syndrome, which is common, was described by Davidson and Wasserman in a useful study of 186 affected children. The symptoms are unexplained chronic or recurrent mild diarrhoea in well thriving children aged one to three. The mother may say that any fruit 'passes right through him'. It is unaffected by dietary treatment or medicine. Mucus is sometimes seen in the stools. There was no evidence of malabsorption or of infection. The authors thought that it resembled the irritable colon of adults.

Certain chronic infections, such as *moniliasis, giardiasis*, and *salmonella* may cause chronic diarrhoea. All are rare in Britain. Monilia would be seen on microscopy. A fresh warm specimen of stool must be examined for giardiasis. The salmonella organisms would be found on culture.

Ulcerative colitis is not rare in children and numerous papers have been written about it. It may begin in the earliest infancy, but it is more common later. It presents with diarrhoea, with blood and mucus in the stool, abdominal pain, associated weight loss and defective physical growth. There may be occasional fever with a poor appetite. Complications include clubbing of the fingers, arthritis, anaemia, stomatitis, other vitamin deficiencies and sometimes hepatic enlargement. The diarrhoea may decrease when milk protein is excluded from the diet (Taylor & Truelove, 1961). Diagnosis is established by sigmoidoscopy and by a barium enema for the typical 'drainpipe' colon with absence of haustration. Crohn's disease of the colon or granulomatous colitis is similar, but the rectum is more likely to be normal on proctoscopy. It may present an unexplained fever, arthritis, erythema nodosum or uveitis before diarrhoea develops.

Appendicitis and intussusception are sometimes associated with diarrhoea (pp. 102, 104), especially if the appendix is pelvic, retrocaecal or retroileal.

A *ganglioneuroma* may cause diarrhoea and failure to thrive.

Thyrotoxicosis or *thyroid overdosage in cretinism* may cause diarrhoea and tremors.

Adrenocortical hyperplasia may present with diarrhoea and dehydration.

Conclusion

When an infant develops acute diarrhoea it should be regarded as a medical emergency. Too often the symptom is treated lightly, the rapidity with which serious and even lethal dehydration may develop being forgotten. When in any doubt the infant should be referred to a hospital for appropriate rehydration by intravenous drip.

When there is chronic looseness of the stools, the child should be referred to a specialist for investigation.

References

BERG I. & JONES K.V. (1964) Functional faecal incontinence in children. *Arch. Dis. Childh.*, **39**, 465.

CORNBLATH M. & SCHWARTZ R. (1966) *Disorders of Carbohydrate Metabolism in Infancy*. Philadelphia, Saunders.

DAVIDSON M. & WASSERMAN R. (1966) The Irritable Colon of Childhood (chronic non-specific diarrhoea). *J. Pediat.*, **69**, 1027.

KORELITZ B.I., GRIBETZ D. & KOPEL F.B. (1968) Granulomatous colitis in children: Study of 25 cases and comparison with ulcerative colitis. *Pediatrics*, **42**, 446.

TAYLOR K.B. & TRUELOVE S.C. (1961) Circulating antibodies to milk protein in ulcerative colitis. *Brit. med. J.*, **2**, 924.

VOORHESS M.L. (1966) Functioning neural tumours. *Pediat. Clinics. N. Amer.*, **13**, 3.

Encopresis and faecal incontinence

Soiling, faecal incontinence, or encopresis, is usually associated with constipation. The mother's complaint is commonly that the child has diarrhoea with soiling, and on rectal examination it is found that the rectum is loaded with a huge mass of faeces. The 'diarrhoea' is due to liquid material leaking round the edge of the faecal mass. When the encopresis is not associated with constipation, it is often accompanied by urinary incontinence. Encopresis is more common in boys than girls. The common age for it is seven to eight years. About half of all affected children have never controlled the bowel, but half have acquired the encopresis, usually as a result of an emotional disturbance, such as the birth of a sibling, starting school, or separation from the mother. The subject was well reviewed by Bellman (1966) and Woodmansey (1967). Encopresis is not a feature of Hirschsprung's disease. Faecal or urinary incontinence may be due to a gross neurological abnormality, such as meningomyelocele or a lipoma involving the spinal cord and is a common feature of mental deficiency.

References

BELLMAN M. (1966) Studies on Encopresis. *Acta Paed. Scand.*, Suppl. 170.
WOODMANSEY A.C. (1967) Emotion and the Motions: an inquiry into the causes and prevention of functional disorders of defaecation. *Brit. J. Med. Psychol.*, **40, 207.**

Blood in the stool

When a newborn baby passes blood in the stool or vomits blood it is essential to determine whether it is the mother's blood or his own (p. 45). If it is the baby's blood, it is a manifestation of haemorrhagic disease of the newborn and arises from some point in the upper part of the alimentary tract, such as the oesophagus. If the baby is breast fed, the blood may have come from the mother's cracked nipple. It is urgent to make the correct diagnosis in order that the appropriate treatment may be given, such as a transfusion.

Blood in the stool of an infant may be due to injury by a rectal thermometer. It is unwise to take the temperature by this route. Blood in the stool of an ill newborn baby may be due to mesenteric thrombosis or perforation of the intestine. The baby will be collapsed, pale and have abdominal distension. There is usually blood in the stool. If the stool is lined with blood, the source is commonly low in the tract. When there is red blood in a baby's stool, the source may be fairly high, while red blood in the stool of an older child would suggest a low source.

The following are conditions to consider in infants and children after the newborn period:

Constipation
Anal fissure
Swallowed blood
Dysentery and salmonella
Ulcerative colitis and Crohn's disease
Milk allergy
Intussusception
Hiatus hernia
Aspirin and other drugs
Peptic ulcer
Hookworm
Meckel's diverticulum
Rare
    Mesenteric thrombosis
    Duplication of the intestine
    Haemangioma of the intestine: telangiectasia
    Rectal polypi
    Blood diseases
    Uraemia
    Haemolytic Uraemic syndrome

After the newborn period, the commonest cause of blood in the stool is *constipation*. This is certainly true if the stools are hard. The blood is found on the outside of the stool. There may or may not be an anal fissure.

Melaena may be due to *swallowed blood*, resulting from an epistaxis or similar cause.

If there is diarrhoea, the usual causes of blood in the stool are infection by *dysentery* or *salmonella*. The diagnosis can be established by culture of the stool. Another cause may be *ulcerative colitis*. This can commence at any age, including the earliest infancy. For this condition and Crohn's disease, see pp. 12 and 82.

If the infant had rhythmical attacks of screaming from abdominal pain, and was pale with shock, blood in the stool would suggest *intussusception* (see p. 104). Chronic intussusception is more easily missed. It is associated with intermittent abdominal pain with blood and mucus in the stool. One may be able to feel the sausage-shaped tumour in the abdomen. The diagnosis can be established by a barium enema.

The quantity of blood in the stool when there is a *hiatus hernia* is small, and unlikely to be detected by any but chemical tests. Blood arising from *oesophageal varices* is more likely to be vomited, but some is likely to pass into the stomach and intestines.

Bleeding from a *peptic ulcer* may occur, but is unusual. Bleeding may result from hookworm infection.

When there is bleeding from a *Meckel's diverticulum*, there is usually little pain. The blood passed is usually dark red. The diagnosis is established by laparotomy. There is an association between Meckel's diverticulum and Turner's syndrome.

Duplication of the intestine may cause considerable blood loss. The diagnosis is usually made by a barium study, but sometimes by laparotomy.

A *haemangioma of the intestine* may cause bleeding from the bowel. Blood loss may result from *intestinal telangiectasia*, and the face should be examined for that condition. It is sometimes associated with blue naevi (blue bleb syndrome), and the skin should be searched for this (Rook *et al.* 1968).

Rectal polyp, or polyp higher in the alimentary tract, may cause considerable bleeding. Rectal polypi can only occasionally be felt by the finger. They are usually found by proctoscopy or sigmoidoscopy. Higher polypi are found by means of a barium enema or laparotomy.

Profuse bleeding from the bowel may occur in the various *blood diseases*, such as thrombocytopenia, allergic purpura or leukaemia. It also occurs in *uraemia*, and in the early stage of the *haemolytic-uraemic* syndrome.

Tests for occult blood in the stool

The family doctor can himself test for occult blood in the stool. Some tests are more sensitive than others; they were reviewed by Ross (1964). The orthotoluidine, 30 second hemastix, and occultest is too sensitive; but if negative, it should exclude bleeding. The child must be on a meat and vegetable free diet for three days before the test is carried out. The hematest tablet test and the 15 second hemastix is not sensitive enough; no special diet is necessary; a positive should mean that blood is present.

A positive test may be due to the child's gums bleeding after brushing the teeth, or to his sucking his finger after a blood test.

References

NADER P.R. & MARGOLIN F. (1966) Hemangioma causing gastrointestinal bleeding. *Am. J. Dis. Child.*, **111**, 215.
ROOK A., WILKINSON D.S. & EBLING F.J.G. (1968) *Textbook of Dermatology.* Oxford, Blackwell Scientific Publications.
ROSS G. & GRAY C.H. (1964) Occult blood tests. *Brit. med. J.*, **1**, 1351.
RUTHERFORD R.B. (1966) Meckel's diverticulum; a review of 148 paediatric patients with special reference to the pattern of bleeding and to meso-diverticular bands. *Surgery*, **59**, 618.

The colour of the stools

The following are the principal colour changes in stools:

Black
  Meconium
  Altered blood
  Iron, bismuth, lead
  Possibly liquorice
  Charcoal
  Eating earth or coal

Abnormally pale
  Obstructive jaundice, including infective hepatitis
  Steatorrhoea
  Aluminium hydroxide
  The periodic syndrome. Stools are often pale in the attacks
Green
  Breast feeding. It is normal for the stools of fully breast fed babie
      to be bright green in colour at times. They may be greei
      when passed, or become green on standing
  Diarrhoea
Red
  Blood
  Viprynium (for threadworms)
  Red gelatin desserts

Pain—some general comments

When we attempt to assess the significance and severity of pain o
what we think is pain, we have to face the difficulty of assessing
someone else's pain. In fact we can only assess it by inference.

The infant shows that he has pain by crying. There are many
causes of crying other than pain, and many an infant is thought to
have pain when he has no such thing. The fact that he draws hi
legs up and cries does not mean that he has pain, for babies usuall
'draw up their legs' when they cry for any reason. I have had
numerous babies referred to me on account of 'acute indigestion
and 'terrible wind', which was supposed to be the reason for the
cries in the night, when in fact the crying was due entirely to the
usual causes of sleep problems—mainly bad habit formation and
parental anxiety. Infants may rub their ears when they have ear
ache, or roll their head or hold it when they have a headache, but
infants rub the ear, roll the head or hold the head when they have
no pain there at all. It may be difficult to decide whether the infan
has pain or not. Severe pain causes a child to emit particularly high

pitched screams. No infant has severe pain if the crying stops as soon as he is picked up.

When the child is old enough to express his feelings in words, it is easier to decide whether he really feels pain. Even so, one has to assess the severity of his pain not by what he says, or even entirely on what the mother says about the pain, but by associated signs. For instance, a pain is not likely to be severe if it does not stop him playing, if it does not stop him eating, if it does not keep him awake, or if there is no change in his colour. A severe pain usually makes the child cry, though some children are more stoical than others. A severe abdominal pain is likely to make the child double up. *It is always profitable to ask the mother whether she would know that he had the pain if he did not tell her that he had it. If she would not know, the pain is not severe.*

We have to assess the child's pain not only by the presence or absence of associated signs, but by our assessment of the mother's personality. The question of whether or not the child is taken to the doctor on account of his pain depends on the parental threshold for anxiety. Some loving mothers will take the child to the doctor if he has the most trivial and short lasting pain; others take the child to the doctor only when the pain is really severe and frequent. Some mothers greatly aggravate a child's pain by displaying anxiety about it, by rubbing his abdomen, petting him and giving him pleasant warm drinks, so that he complains all the more as an attention-seeking device. In fact, in order to assess a child's pain, one has to assess the family pattern of behaviour as a whole and to determine whether other members of the family have similar pains. This is not merely because migraine or peptic ulcer commonly has a hereditary basis; it is because a child may imitate his parents, consciously or unconsciously, or fear that he has the same symptoms. If his father frequently complains about his gastric symptoms, or has had to go to hospital on their account, or if the mother is seen to have incapacitating attacks of migraine, it would not be surprising if the child also experienced pains, not necessarily due directly to peptic ulcer or migraine. When talking to a child about pain, it is important to ask whether any of his friends have a similar pain. The answer is frequently in the affirmative.

A child may experience pain (particularly in the head or abdomen) as a result of worries and anxieties about school. He may be in difficulty with a particular subject such as arithmetic, or he may be worried by a teacher's loud voice or threats of punishment. He may be worried because of bullying or because of teasing about his clothes, his appearance, his obesity. He may experience the pain when he is getting ready to go to school. He is not necessarily malingering; he is not pretending: he may really experience the pain, though it is entirely psychological in origin.

Pain may be suggested by an anxious mother. A few minutes after I had talked to a mother about her boy's abdominal pain, telling her that I had found no disease to explain it, she was overheard saying to the boy, 'Of course you have pain in your tummy, darling, haven't you?' He had.

Headache

Headache is a common symptom in childhood. Apley at Bristol found that one in seven children of school age complained of headache. Vahlquist in Sweden found that 4.5 per cent of 1236 children had migraine, and a further 13.3 per cent had other forms of headache. Oster and Nielsen found that 20.6 per cent of 2178 school children experienced headaches. Yet nine popular textbooks of paediatrics (in 14 volumes) contained a total of only $1\frac{1}{4}$ pages on the subject, and six of these popular textbooks do not include headache in the index.

In not more than five per cent of children referred to hospital on account of headache is any organic cause discovered.

The following are the main conditions which should be considered:

Psychological factors
Infection
Physical environmental factors
  a stuffy room
  lack of fresh air
  climatic conditions (e.g., thunder)

Hunger
Migraine
Epilepsy
Head injury
Intracranial causes
Osteitis
Nephritis
Hypertension
Benign Intracranial Hypertension
Effect of drugs
Earache or toothache
Eye strain (rare). Glaucoma
Antrum infection (rare)
Basilar impression syndrome (rare)

A variety of *psychological factors* are associated with headaches. They include worry and anxiety about school work, about an unkind teacher or about bullying. There is the well-known 'headache of convenience' which may bring about a happy release from the arithmetic class. A headache may well become an attention-seeking device if excessive anxiety is shown about it. For the combination of headaches and growing pains, see p. 226.

Any infection may be accompanied at its onset by a headache and by non-specific aches and pains. Amongst less obvious infective causes of headaches or general lassitude is an apical tooth infection.

Simple factors such as *hunger*, a *stuffy room*, *lack of fresh air and exercise*, an *impending thunderstorm*, may be important and common causes of headache. It may be due to hunger and hypoglycaemia.

Migraine is a common symptom of childhood. I do not think that one can draw a clear-cut line between migraine and other headaches, though for research purposes, such as the assessment of a drug, one would define migraine as typically a unilateral headache with vomiting, preceded by visual aurae and having a hereditary basis, but the pain is by no means always unilateral. A comprehensive review of childhood migraine, running into 147 pages, was written by Bille (1962).

Symptoms of migraine commonly begin in early childhood. Vomiting attacks which recur and which later turn out to be due to migraine may begin as early as six months of age. In at least a third of all children with migraine symptoms begin before the fourth year. Selby & Lance (1960) found that 30 per cent of their 500 cases of migraine began before the age of ten.

Migraine may manifest itself in childhood by any combination of the following symptoms—headache, vomiting, abdominal pain or fever, sometimes associated with the passage of pale stools. This group of symptoms is commonly termed the 'periodic syndrome'. It used to be termed 'cyclical vomiting' or 'acidosis attacks' until it was realised that the acidosis was the result of the attacks, and not their cause. There may be premonitory visual, sensory or mental symptoms, the commonest visual aura consisting of fortification figures. There may be aphasia, blurring of vision or paraesthesiae in the limbs. Sometimes these symptoms occur without a headache. It is said that a convulsion can occur during the premonitory phase. The headache is commonly described as unilateral and frontal, and some would not accept the diagnosis of migraine otherwise; but I disagree with this rigid view of migraine. Selby & Lance, in their analysis of 500 cases of migraine, found that 38 per cent had hemicrania alone (and that in 21 per cent the headache was always on the same side), 23 per cent had hemicrania and general headache, and 38 per cent had pain all over the head. It is interesting to note that there was no difference with regard to the incidence and nature of associated phenomena between those with hemicrania and those with general headache. The attacks may last an hour or two, or two or three days. They commonly last a few hours, and are relieved by sleep.

The initial symptoms are associated with vasoconstriction of the intracranial arteries, leading to the visual and other symptoms, with marked pallor, followed by dilatation of the vessels with the development of a headache which is commonly throbbing in character. Later there may be suffusion of the face and conjunctivae and even a haematoma.

Bille and others considered that children who suffer from migraine are more likely to be shy, anxious, sensitive and more vulnerable to frustration than controls; their parents tend to be more perfectionist, rigid, ambitious and efficient than others. The attacks tend to be precipitated by fatigue, anxiety, excitement, conflict at home or school, noise or exposure to bright light, including the television screen. They may be related to menstruation or follow an infection. Hunger may bring on an attack. It is often said that allergy may be a factor. Attacks may be precipitated by cheese and other milk products, chocolates or broad beans.

The diagnosis is not always easy. There are no pathognomonic signs of migraine. Apparently typical attacks of migraine may be due to an intracranial aneurism. One is particularly concerned about this possibility when a child has neurological signs in the attacks—such as aphasia, paraesthesiae or weakness of a limb. It is essential to include ophthalmoscopy in one's examination, together with a blood pressure estimation to exclude hypertension. It is a matter of experienced clinical judgment to decide at what stage further investigation is required. The necessary investigation would include carotid angiography, a procedure not without risk, for up to one per cent subjected to this investigation may develop a hemiplegia. An ophthalmologist referred a 12-year-old girl to me on account of migraine, having found that she had no abnormality on examination of the eyes. The history was typical of migraine and there was a family history of the same complaint. There were no abnormal physical signs, but there was considerable psychological instability. I discussed the diagnosis with the parents, telling them that the girl had migraine. Three days later, on an excursion to the seaside, the girl slowly and imperceptibly lapsed into unconsciousness. A carotid angiogram did not show any abnormality, but a vertebral angiogram showed an aneurism of the vertebral artery. Cerebral tumours can for a time give a picture identical with that of migraine.

There is an important danger in the diagnosis of recurrent attacks of migraine. A child may have several attacks of migraine, and then unfortunately develop pyogenic meningitis with similar symptoms. The true diagnosis may then be missed.

There are occasions when it is necessary to distinguish migraine from *epilepsy*. The latter condition may manifest itself by sudden attacks of severe headache of instantaneous onset lasting for a few minutes followed by sleep, but without convulsive phenomena. Many children go to sleep in an attack of migraine. It has already been stated that during the phase of vasoconstriction in the intra-cranial vessels, a convulsion may occur. The aura of migraine may lead to the wrong diagnosis of epilepsy—though an aura is defin-itely unusual in childhood epilepsy. When in doubt an electro-encephalogram should be carried out, though an EEG is often normal in epilepsy of grand mal type and so may not help. One is then justified in carrying out the therapeutic test of giving pheny-toin in full dosage; it should stop the attacks if they are epileptic in origin.

In 70 or 80 per cent of cases of migraine there is a family history of the same complaint, though headaches in adults are common, whether or not their children have migraine. If there is anything about the story of the child's attacks which raises a doubt in my mind about the diagnosis, I would be more doubtful if there were no history of migraine in the parents.

Follow-up studies following *head injuries* have shown how rarely head injury in children is followed by sequelae—except in the case of severe head injury with laceration of the brain. The ordi-nary mild concussion, so common in children, is most unlikely to be followed by headaches in subsequent weeks and months, and if they do occur, they are much more likely to be related to heredity or environmental and personality factors than to the injury. In the same way emotional sequelae of head injuries are more likely to be related to previous personality traits and subse-quent environmental factors than to any structural defect resulting from the injury (Otto, 1960). Nevertheless, when one sees any child complaining of headache following a head injury, one must ex-amine the optic fundi for papilloedema, indicating increased intra-cranial pressure, and it is wise to have an x-ray of the skull taken, if it has not already been done, in case there has been a fracture. An EEG may also be performed, for this may indicate the possi-bility of a subdural haematoma. In an infant serial head circum-ference measurements must be taken, in order to help to exclude a subdural haematoma. Bulging of the fontanelle or undue separation of the sutures may also be found. If in doubt, the specialist will carry out subdural taps.

Other *intracranial causes* of headache include *tumour, abscess, arteriovenous malformations, poliomyelitis, encephalitis and menin-*

gitis. Normal optic discs, though not excluding a space occupying lesion, help to make such a lesion unlikely. Osteitis of the skull would be obvious on simple examination.

The nature of the headache is of some value in diagnosis. An occipital headache is more likely to be due to an organic lesion than a frontal one, though a supratentorial tumour commonly causes a frontal headache. The headache of increased intracranial pressure is liable to be affected by change of posture; it is worse on rising in the morning, on stooping or on straining. It is apt to be a dull, throbbing or bursting pain, while a headache of nervous origin is more likely to consist of a feeling of pressure; but the headache of migraine may be of a throbbing nature.

Apart from ophthalmoscopic examination, which can never be omitted from the examination of a child with headache, one must remember to auscultate the skull, because that might lead to the diagnosis of an intracranial vascular anomaly. When an infant is being examined because of the possibility of a cerebral tumour, the skull should be percussed. A 'cracked pot sound' may be elicited if there is increased intracranial tension. One may also be able to detect undue separation of the cranial sutures.

Nephritis and *hypertension* are possible causes of headache. It follows that the examination cannot be complete without examination of the urine for nephritis and pyelonephritis, and without recording the blood pressure. Rose and Matson (1967) reviewed the condition of *benign intracranial hypertension*, describing 23 cases. There was a sudden onset of headache with sixth nerve palsy and papilloedema without loss of consciousness. The C.S.F. was normal. In some cases there was a preceding respiratory infection, otitis media or head injury. Recovery was complete. The condition may follow discontinuation of corticosteroid therapy. It occurs with overdosage of vitamin A, hypovitaminosis A, hypoparathyroidism, the use of tetracyclines or ampicillin and in blood diseases.

Pain from an *ear or a tooth* may cause a headache.

Eyestrain is a most unlikely cause of headache, unless the symptom of eyestrain is obvious. If the child cannot see his book without bringing his eyes very close to it, or if he cannot read what is written on the blackboard, then his eyes should be tested. Ophthalmoscopic examination is a routine part of the examination of any child with a headache. If the fundi are normal, and in the absence of any symptom pointing to the eyes, the child's visit to the eye specialist is most unlikely to be profitable. Glaucoma is a rare cause.

A chronic antrum infection is most unlikely to be a cause of recurrent headaches. I do not think that I have ever seen a case of headache due to a chronic infection of the antrum. In any case, a chronic antrum infection can be diagnosed with reasonable certainty on clinical grounds. There will be a history of a continuous purulent discharge between colds, or of a continual postnasal discharge, visible on examination of the throat, and causing the usual symptoms, such as cough on lying down and constant clearing of the throat. An x-ray of the antrum will confirm the diagnosis. In my experience children with a chronic infection are no more likely to suffer from headaches than any other child. It is obvious that an acute antrum infection may cause a headache.

A variety of drugs may cause headaches: they include acetazolamide, amitriptyline, antihistamines, chlorpromazine, diazepam, ephedrine, ethosuccimide, griseofulvin, indomethacin, methylphenidate, nalidixic acid, nitrofurantoin, paromomycin, phenytoin, rifampicin, sulphasalazine, sulphonamides, sulthiame, tetracycline, thiobendazole, trimethoprim, troxidone and vincristine.

Lead poisoning may cause headaches. The *basilar impression syndrome* causes persistent occipital headache. There is a short neck, lower cranial nerve palsy, nystagmus, ataxia or spasticity. It is due to a congenital abnormality of the upper cervical spine and base of the skull. It may be associated with the Klippel–Feil syndrome.

Because of the ever-present possibility of a serious organic cause every child presenting with a headache demands careful history taking and a full general and neurological examination, including ophthalmoscopy. If a child is completely well between the attacks, he is much less likely to have serious organic disease than if there were a complaint of lassitude, loss of appetite, loss of weight or the development of clumsiness of movement; all these symptoms would strongly suggest a serious organic disease.

References

Bille B. (1962) Migraine in school children. *Acta Paediat. Uppsala*, Suppl. 136, 51.

Friedman A. & Harms F. (1967) *Headaches in Children.* Charles Thomas.
Grant D.N. (1971) Benign intracranial hypertension. *Arch. Dis. Childh.,* **46,** 651.
Hagberg B. & Sillinpaa M. (1970) Benign intracranial hypertension: review and report of 18 cases. *Acta Paediat. Scandinav.,* **59,** 328.
Oster J. & Nielsen A. (1972) Growing Pains. *Acta Paediat. Scandinav.,* **61,** 329.
Otto U. (1960) Postconcussion syndrome. *Acta paedopsychiatrica,* **1,** 6.
Selby G. & Lance J.W. (1960) Observations on 500 cases of migraine and allied vascular headaches. *J. Neurol. Neurosurg. Psychiat.,* **23,** 23.

Abdominal pain

Non-organic causes of abdominal pain in the infant

The commonest causes of abdominal pain in an infant who is not ill are *wind* and *evening colic.* Excessive wind has been discussed elsewhere (p. 67).

Evening colic, also called three months' colic, is a somewhat mysterious condition which affects well thriving babies, breast fed or artificially fed, in the first two or three months after birth. It commences within a week or two of birth with abdominal pain, mainly in the evening between 6.0 p.m. and 10.0 p.m. The pain may be mild, causing the baby to be restless, or severe, causing rhythmical screaming attacks, lasting a few minutes, alternating with quiet periods in which the baby almost goes to sleep. In the attacks loud borborygmi can be heard and the child obtains some relief in the prone position or on passing flatus per rectum. It is prevented by an anti-cholinergic drug, dicyclomine hydrochloride (one teaspoonful of the liquid), before the evening feed. It is probable that the pain is due to wind becoming locked in a loop of bowel.

Acute abdominal pain

The history

A careful detailed history is an essential step to the diagnosis. In the first place, one needs to know how long the child has had the pain, asking in particular whether he ever had it before the date mentioned, and whether before that date he was in all respects perfectly well.

One next needs to know whether the pain is continuous or intermittent. If it is intermittent, one needs to know how frequent the attacks are, how long they last, and whether they are becoming more or less frequent. One frequently finds that the pain is infrequent—for example once in three or four months, and that when it occurs it only lasts for a minute or two. This is important, because one has to try to assess the significance of the complaint. In the case of an acute abdominal pain, it is usually true to say that a pain which comes and goes is unlikely to be due to appendicitis, the pain of which is more often continuous.

One needs to know where the pain is. Most of the non-organic recurrent abdominal pains of childhood are localised vaguely in the umbilical region. Apley remarked that the further the pain is localised away from the umbilicus, the more likely is there to be an underlying organic disorder. I would feel that when a child complains of pain in one part of the body one day and a different part on another, and there is no constant localisation, organic disease is less likely than when the pain is always localised to one area. An obvious exception to this is the pain of acute appendicitis, which may begin in the umbilical region and settle later in the right iliac fossa.

There are not many examples of referred pain in children. The most common is the pain of pleurisy, as in lobar pneumonia. Pleurisy over the right lower lobe is referred to the right iliac fossa, and pleurisy over the left lower lobe to the left iliac fossa. Severe pain may be felt in the upper abdomen when the upper part of the pleura is involved. Pain in the knee may originate from inflammation or other disease in the hip, being referred by the obturator nerve. Pain in the tip of the left shoulder may originate from a ruptured spleen (e.g. in a sledging accident).

The severity of the pain has to be assessed. Zachary (1965) suggested that one should ask the child 'whether it is different from ordinary tummy-ache'. Apley found that a quarter of the children with recurrent abdominal pain without organic disease suffered from severe pain. He wrote that the truly severe pain, causing the child to thresh and writhe in agony, is hardly ever organic in origin.

Whether the pain is continuous or intermittent, one must determine whether the pain is getting better or worse. One pays more attention to a pain which is becoming worse.

The nature of the pain may be helpful in diagnosis. A stabbing pain, feeling as if needles are being pushed in, may be pleural or peritoneal in origin. A pain which regularly comes and goes, lasting for a minute or two, with corresponding free intervals, suggests an alimentary origin. Bouts of pain in an ill child would make the diagnosis of acute appendicitis most unlikely.

The mode of onset may be important. A pain of instantaneous onset lasting a few minutes only and followed by sleep may be due to epilepsy. The duration of the pain is important. *An attack of abdominal pain lasting more than three hours should be regarded as an abdominal emergency until proved otherwise.*

It may be useful to ask what brings the pain on, what relieves it and what makes it worse. A pleural pain (and sometimes a peritoneal pain) is worse on breathing or coughing.

It is vital to enquire about associated symptoms. An associated headache may point to migraine, though headache may be a symptom of fever due to any cause. Associated diarrhoea suggests an alimentary origin. Associated urinary symptoms suggest a lesion of the urinary tract. In the case of an acute abdominal pain, associated vomiting should indicate the need for great caution in the diagnosis, for it may well point to a condition for which surgical treatment will be needed. When the pain is due to an acute surgical condition, it usually precedes other symptoms, such as vomiting (Zachary, 1965).

Finally one must assess the family as a whole. One must know whether other members of the family have abdominal pains. One must assess the personality of the parents, note whether they are tense, anxious, worried or placid characters, for this will help one to establish the diagnosis.

The examination

When a child presents with abdominal pain, the whole child must be examined, if for no other reason but the fact that many extra-abdominal conditions cause pain in the abdomen.

Many a small child steadfastly refuses to lie down when asked to do, and determined efforts to get him to lie down will inevitably lead to tears, so that it becomes impossible to examine the abdomen adequately. In fact it is reasonably satisfactory to examine the child's abdomen when he is standing up or kneeling. Sometimes it is impossible to get the child to relax, and in that case, if accurate examination is vital, he should be given a sedative such as rectal barbiturate or intramuscular paraldehyde. Even if the child is crying, increased vigour of crying may help to localise the site of pain and tenderness.

Medical students commonly make the mistake of keeping the eyes on the abdomen when palpating it. I commonly tell them that omphaloscopy does not help in establishing the diagnosis. It is essential to watch the child's face in order to detect signs of abdominal tenderness. Another common mistake is to examine the abdomen when the head is elevated on two or more pillows. Unless the head is flat on the bed, or only slightly elevated on a low pillow (which is often preferable), it may be impossible to detect splenic enlargement.

Tenderness over the descending colon is not of importance. There may be only deep tenderness when an inflamed appendix is retrocaecal. Rectal examination is essential in any child with acute abdominal pain. One notes particularly whether there is more tenderness or heat on one side than on the other. Inspection of the hernial orifices must not be omitted.

Auscultation of the abdomen may contribute to the diagnosis of ileus, the absence of peristaltic sounds being the important feature of that condition.

The diagnosis

Joseph Brennemann, famous Chicago paediatrician, wrote as follows: 'After 40 years of extensive experience I still approach the acutely painful abdomen of a child with much apprehension and a greater feeling of uncertainty than any other domain of childhood.'

The cause of the pain may be nothing more than a dietary indiscretion: but there are many more important causes, which will be outlined below.

The following are the main conditions which should be considered:

Pain from vomiting, coughing, or diarrhoea

Lobar pneumonia and pleurisy, pleurodynia, other respiratory tract infections

Appendicitis

Acute peritonitis

Mesenteric lymphadenitis

Intussusception

Intestinal obstruction, including strangulated hernia and volvulus

Fibrocystic disease of the pancreas

Roundworms

Urinary tract infection

Acute nephritis

Renal colic

Infective hepatitis

Cholecystitis

Diabetes, diabetic acidosis, hypoglycaemia

Anaphylactoid purpura (p. 54)

Rheumatic fever

Rare

    Pancreatitis

    Rupture of the spleen

    Regional ileitis (p. 12)

    Zollinger-Ellison syndrome (p. 76)

    Meckel's diverticulitis

    Twisted ovarian pedicle or ruptured ovarian cyst

    Torsion of the testis

    Crises of sickle cell anaemia

    Lead poisoning (pp. 51, 96)

    Glandular fever

    Drugs

    Acute infectious lymphocytosis

    Porphyria

    Haemophilia

Pain from vomiting, diarrhoea, or coughing. Any child with severe vomiting or coughing may experience some abdominal pain.

Lobar pneumonia and pleurisy. Referred pain from pleurisy with or without pneumonia is a common source of confusion in a child with acute abdominal pain. The finding of reduced air entry at one base, possibly with a slight alteration in the character of the breath sounds, or the so-called indux crepitations, should indicate lobar pneumonia. An x-ray of the chest confirms the diagnosis. Pleural friction may be heard if there is pneumonia and pleurisy. *Epidemic pleurodynia* (Bornholm disease) may give rise to severe abdominal pain.

Abdominal pain may be a complaint when a child has *tonsillitis* or other respiratory tract infection, including measles. Sometimes this may be due to mesenteric lymphadenitis (below).

Appendicitis

The symptoms and signs of appendicitis are so well known that I do not propose to describe them here. Instead I shall draw attention to the common sources of error in diagnosis. In an excellent paper, Jackson of Newcastle (1963) described many of these sources of confusion. These are as follows:

(1) The appendix is not always in the 'typical' position. Of Jackson's 313 cases in childhood, the appendix was in the typical site in 32 per cent, retrocaecal in 27 per cent, pelvic in 23 per cent, and elsewhere (retroileal, subhepatic, splenic, or left iliac fossa) in 11 per cent. When the appendix is retrocaecal there may be no abdominal tenderness.

(2) It is only in some 30 per cent of cases that the pain begins in the periumbilical region and then settles in the right iliac fossa. In some 20 per cent the pain is confined to the central area, in 25 per cent it is confined to the right iliac fossa, whereas in the remaining 25 per cent it is situated elsewhere in the abdomen.

(3) Though the pain of appendicitis is usually continuous from the onset, it is occasionally intermittent. It was intermittent throughout in 12 per cent of Jackson's cases, and in a further 22 per cent it was intermittent first and continuous later.

(4) The pain may be mild or even absent. In four of Jackson's 313 cases there was no complaint of pain at all. Mildness of the pain may well lead to delay in diagnosis.

(5) There is not always vomiting.

(6) There may be urinary symptoms and signs, particularly in children in whom the appendix is in the pelvis. Above 12 per cent experience some dysuria. There may be an excess of white blood cells in the urine.

(7) Instead of the usual constipation there may be diarrhoea. About ten per cent experience this symptom, which may cause serious confusion in the diagnosis. Diarrhoea is especially liable to occur when the appendix is pelvic, retrocaecal or retroileal.

(8) Though the temperature is not usually high, about five per cent have a temperature of over 39°C.

(9) Appendicitis is rare under the age of three (though it can occur in early infancy), and when it does occur the diagnosis may well be missed. Howard Williams of Melbourne described 42 cases in this age group. He found that 50 per cent presented an abdominal mass due to perforation; 37 per cent presented with general peritonitis; 20 per cent had diarrhoea; and eight per cent had dysuria. The symptoms were fever, vomiting, fretfulness and diarrhoea. Another Australian, Auldist (1967), reviewed 203 cases of appendicitis under the age of five years. He found anorexia in 99 per cent, vomiting in 94 per cent, pain in 93 per cent, fever in 58 per cent, respiratory symptoms in 31 per cent, and diarrhoea and constipation each in 26 per cent. In 38 per cent there was a palpable mass in the right iliac fossa.

(10) Previous attacks of abdominal pain. In about one in every ten cases of acute appendicitis, there is a history of previous attacks of pain. Recurrent attacks of abdominal pain favour the diagnosis of a non-organic cause.

(11) Appendicitis may coexist with other conditions, notably acute tonsillitis, but also with pneumonia, urinary tract infection or even gastroenteritis.

Acute peritonitis should be considered when a child is acutely ill with abdominal pain and fever, and generalised rigidity is found on abdominal examination. The commonest cause of peritonitis is a perforated appendix, but the peritonitis may be due to the pneumo coccus or other pyogenic organism. Holgersen and Stanley-Brown (1971), analysing 100 cases of acute appendicitis with perforation found that vomiting, fever and abdominal pain were the main symptoms, but in 40 per cent there was an unlocalised abdominal pain, and in five per cent there was no pain at all. In one child the pain was confined to the testis. Four had had previous abdominal pain. The white cell was not helpful in infancy, eight infants having a white cell count of less than 10,000. In 28 there was albuminuria in nine haematuria, and in 16 acetonuria. There was a significant increase of white cells in the urine of 24 children.

Mesenteric lymphadenitis. This may be difficult to distinguish from acute appendicitis. It is said that a shifting of the point of maximum tenderness on turning the patient on his side is in favour of mesenteric adenitis. It is not a reliable sign. The temperature tends to be higher in mesenteric adenitis than in appendicitis, but it is not always so. There may be a tonsillitis in either case. There is usually more true rigidity over the right iliac fossa in a child with acute appendicitis. When in doubt, which is not infrequent, one will establish the diagnosis by laparotomy.

Intussusception

The common age at which intussusception occurs is five to nine months. It is unusual after the first two years. It is said to be more common in babies who are above the average weight and who are artificially fed. Intussusception should be strongly suspected when an infant becomes suddenly ill with abdominal pain, vomiting and pallor. The most common initial symptom is pain, and vomiting usually follows shortly after. The onset may be so sudden that the mother may be able to state the exact time at which the pain started. The pain is commonly rhythmical in character, coming and going. The child characteristically becomes pale in each spasm. He rapidly becomes ill, goes off his food, becoming pale and collapsed. In some cases there may be no pain at all, the only sign being sudden collapse with pallor and shock. The colic commonly lasts for two or three minutes, recurring every 15 to 20 minutes. After three or four attacks the child is likely to be pale and drowsy. Intussusception should always be suspected if attacks of colic persist for over two hours. The passage of blood in the stool is not usually an early symptom. A history of previous attacks of abdominal pain is a point in favour of the diagnosis.

On examination in an early case there may be a palpable mass in the right upper quadrant of the abdomen; later there may be a tumour to the left of the midline. The mass is best felt during a spasm of pain. It is most often felt in the right hypochondium but may be felt anywhere along the line of the colon. When in doubt and the child is crying, one palpates the abdomen after a sedative has been given. Even when one cannot feel a mass, there may be guarding over the upper part of the right rectus muscle. On rectal examination the rectum is empty; there may be blood on the finger stall.

Ravitch (1952) described some of the snares which may lead to wrong diagnoses. They are as follows:

(1) Thirty per cent pass a stool in the first 24 hours. This may lead one to think that intestinal obstruction is unlikely.

(2) Seven per cent have diarrhoea at the onset. This, with blood in the stool, leads to an erroneous diagnosis of dysentery.

(3) There may be no blood in the stool. This applies to about a third of cases—at least in the early stage.

(4) There may be no vomiting for 6 to 12 hours.

(5) There is commonly an elevation of temperature. In two-thirds of cases the temperature is over 100°F and in a quarter 102°F or more.

(6) In ten to 20 per cent there is a history of preceding upper respiratory tract infection and there may be a cough.

(7) One in six children has a leucocytosis (20,000 per mm^3 or more). This may suggest that there is nothing more than an infection.

(8) Chronic intussusception may present with a history of days or weeks of abdominal pain, vomiting, constipation and the presence of blood and mucus in the stools. The diagnosis of ulcerative colitis or salmonella infection could easily be made.

The clinical diagnosis is confirmed by a straight x-ray of the abdomen, followed, if necessary, by a barium enema.

Other causes

Children with *fibrocystic disease of the pancreas* may experience attacks of abdominal pain, sometimes as a result of faecal impaction.

In countries abroad *roundworms* may cause attacks of abdominal pain.

Abdominal pain may result from an acute *urinary tract infection*, but it is not a particularly common symptom.

A child at the onset of *acute nephritis* may experience severe pain in the abdomen, which may lead to the diagnosis of appendicitis. Examination of the urine for albumin, red cells and granular and cellular casts will establish the diagnosis.

Renal colic is an unusual cause of abdominal pain in children. It may occur as a result of sulphadiazine crystalluria, or as a result of calculus formation in a child who has been recumbent for a long time.

Infective hepatitis. Some children at the onset of infective hepatitis experience pain in the right upper quadrant of the abdomen. The diagnosis should be established by the presence of bilirubin in the urine and icterus.

Cholecystitis is rare in children. It is accompanied by pain in the right upper quadrant of the abdomen, vomiting, fever and abdominal distension. It is difficult to distinguish from intestinal obstruction or a high retrocaecal appendicitis.

Abdominal pain is an important symptom of *diabetic acidosis* or of *hypoglycaemia*.

At the onset of an attack of *acute rheumatic fever*, there may be severe pain in the right iliac fossa. It is likely that in such a case there would be other signs of rheumatic fever, such as arthritis.

The most common cause of *acute pancreatitis* is mumps. Three or four days after the swelling of the parotid gland there is vomiting, periumbilical abdominal pain, shock and then diarrhoea. There may be fever, bulky stools and polyuria. Acute pancreatitis not due to mumps is accompanied by severe upper abdominal pain, vomiting, shock and distension of the abdomen. The diagnosis is confirmed by a high serum amylase and lipase. There may also be hyperglycaemia, glycosuria and albuminuria.

Pancreatitis may be caused by various *drugs*, including chlorothiazide, corticosteroids, immunosuppressants, indomethacin, isoniazid, salicylates and sulphonamides. The symptoms include abdominal pain, vomiting and a distended upper abdomen. The diagnosis is confirmed by a high serum and urinary amylase.

Ruptured spleen may be associated with pain in the abdomen and pain referred to the left shoulder, with pallor and shock.

Meckel's diverticulitis. This is likely to cause pain in the right iliac fossa. A previous history of blood in the stool, or the presence of blood in the stool in the present attack, would suggest the diagnosis, which can be confirmed conclusively only by laparotomy.

An *ovarian cyst, rupture of ovarian follicles or twisted ovarian pedicle* may cause lower abdominal pain with shock and vomiting.

Torsion of the testis may occur at any time in childhood, from the first day onwards. It is more common in the first year. It causes severe pain, vomiting and shock. The pain often commences in sleep or during exercise: it commonly begins in the inguinal region of the abdomen just above the internal inguinal ring. It is commonly confused with acute epididymitis, but this is exceedingly rare in the absence of a urinary tract infection. It has to be distinguished from orchitis due to mumps and tuberculosis, testicular neoplasm or injury, and haemorrhage in purpura. On occasion there is a scrotal swelling which could be mistaken for orchitis, epididymitis, strangulated hernia or testicular tumour. Treatment is urgent to preserve the testis (Naef, 1961).

Sickle cell anaemia crises in coloured children may cause severe abdominal pain. The diagnosis is made by the haematologist. The pain may be accompanied by rigidity of the abdominal wall, pains in the legs, arthritis, flank pain or convulsions. Jaundice usually follows in two or three days.

Glandular fever and acute infectious lymphocytosis may be associated with abdominal pain.

Pain may be precipitated in *porphyria* by sulphonamides or barbiturates.

Drugs which may cause abdominal pain include amitriptyline, azathiaprine, cephalosporins, chlordiazepoxide, corticosteroids, dichlorophen, erythromycin, ethionamide, gentian violet, imipramine, iodides, iron, lincomycin, methotrexate, nystatin, P.A.S. paromomycin, phenytoin, piperazine, primidone, rifampicin, tetracycline, trimethoprim, troxidone, vincristine and viprynium.

Conclusion

As stated at the beginning of this section, the diagnosis of the cause of acute abdominal pain in a child may be a matter of the greatest difficulty. It is certainly a matter of the utmost importance, and many tragedies are constantly being caused by overconfidence, which so often involves delay in the diagnosis of some condition which could readily have been cured by prompt surgical treatment. It follows that there should be no hesitation in calling in expert advice when one is faced with the problem of a child with acute abdominal pain.

Recurrent abdominal pain

When faced with a child suffering from recurrent abdominal pain, the following conditions should be considered:

Psychological factors
Hydronephrosis
Peptic ulcer
Abdominal epilepsy
Abdominal allergy
Constipation
Worm infestation
Lead poisoning

Psychological factors

In his excellent monograph on *The Child with Abdominal Pains* Apley described a study of 1000 school children in Bristol. The incidence of abdominal pains was 12·3 per cent in girls and 9·5 per cent in boys. In 92 per cent of children referred for recurrent abdominal pain, no organic cause could be found after full investigation. In half of the affected children, there was another member of the family who suffered from pains. Two out of three had associated vomiting, one out of two had pallor in the attacks, and one out of five had headaches. One out of four went to sleep after the attack. Various comparisons were made between affected children and controls. The incidence of appendicectomy was 17 times greater than in controls and headaches were three times more frequent. The incidence of convulsions, however, was three times greater in controls than in the children with abdominal pains. There was a much greater incidence of headaches, nervous breakdowns and other nervous symptoms in the family of affected children than in the family of controls. With regard to the level of intelligence, there was no difference between the affected children and controls. The pain was umbilical in two-thirds; it consisted usually of a dull ache, and in a quarter it was severe. It occurred in the day or night, and occasionally in holidays. The duration and frequency varied considerably from child to child. Of 30 children followed up eight to 12 years later, nine were symptom free and three had migraine.

Complaints of pain may be an attention-seeking device. If the mother expresses anxiety about the child's complaints, rubs his abdomen, gives him sweets, medicine or a warm drink and makes him lie down, the pain is apt to recur.

A child may complain of pain in imitation of one of his parents, who is constantly complaining of his pains. He may feel worried about his parents' symptom and express his anxiety by feeling the same pain as that of his parent. Pains may be due to worry and anxiety—worries about bullying at school, fear of a particular teacher or dislike of being teased. Bayless and Huang (1971) suggested that some cases of recurrent abdominal pain are due to lactose intolerance, and that they respond to removal of milk from the diet.

Hydronephrosis can cause troublesome abdominal pain. The pain is by no means always localised to the loins. It is frequently impossible to palpate the kidney and the urine may be entirely normal on examination. Even if there is a pyonephrosis, the flow of urine from the affected kidney may be blocked, so that the urine examined is normal. One can never entirely eliminate hydronephrosis as a cause of abdominal pain without a pyelogram. Abdominal pains in children are common, and one wants to avoid pyelography where possible for three important reasons: it is unpleasant for the child; it involves a fairly considerable degree of irradiation; and there is a small risk of dangerous iodine sensitivity. One has to use one's judgment, therefore, in deciding whether an intravenous pyelogram is needed. The further danger of a retrograde pyelogram is the introduction of infection by instrumentation. Even if one finds a double renal element as a result of the pyelography, one cannot be sure whether the pain is related to the renal anomaly or not.

There are widely differing views as to the frequency of *peptic ulceration* in children. Some regard it as common while some think that it is rare. Many adults with proved peptic ulcer date the onset of abdominal symptoms to childhood. The symptoms in a child are much more vague and indefinite than they are in an adult. The diagnosis can be made by the finding of occult blood in the stools and by a barium meal examination. The latter involves irradiation and one has to use one's judgment in deciding whether to have it done or not.

Abdominal epilepsy is a possible cause of recurrent abdominal pain. In order to make the diagnosis one must obtain a history that the attacks are of sudden onset, last a few minutes only and are followed by sleep. An electroencephalogram may confirm the diagnosis, but the EEG is frequently normal in epilepsy of grand mal type. The therapeutic test of phenytoin and phenobarbitone in full dosage is perhaps a more reliable method of establishing the diagnosis.

Though some would say that *allergy* is a common cause of abdominal pain, I have seen few children for whom I found this diagnosis satisfactory. Nevertheless, one should ask whether any particular food causes the child's pain. One may then try to prevent the pain by elimination diets.

Constipation is commonly blamed for abdominal pain in children. Unless there is actual impaction of faeces causing intestinal obstruction, I am doubtful whether constipation ever causes abdominal pain in children. It is certain that children with gross constipation, often with soiling, hardly ever suffer from abdominal pain. If they do not have pain, it seems unlikely that children with a much less degree of constipation would have pain either. Davidson (1971) ascribed many recurrent abdominal pains to hypertonus of the colon with excessive drying of the stool and therefore constipation. Kopel *et al.* (1967) had previously expressed a similar view.

Worm infestation with ascaris may cause pain. It is probably rare in Britain. Unless *threadworms* block the appendix, I find it difficult to believe that they would cause pain. I cannot imagine the mechanism whereby minute threads, averaging a few millimetres in length and lying loosely in the intestine would cause abdominal pain.

Unknown causes. Usually there is no discoverable cause for recurrent abdominal pain in otherwise well children.

References

APLEY J. (1959) *The Child with Abdominal Pain*. Oxford, Blackwell Scientific Publications.

AULDIST A.W. (1967) Appendicitis in patients under five years of age. *Australian Paed. J.*, 3, 144.

BAYLESS T.M. & HUANG S.-S. (1971) Recurrent abdominal pain due to milk and lactose intolerance in school aged children. *Pediatrics*, 47, 1029.

CHAPMAN R.H. & WALTON A.J. (1972) Torsion of the testis and its appendages. *Brit. Med. J.*, 1, 164.

DAVIDSON M. (1971) Recurrent abdominal pain. *Am. J. Dis. Child.*, 121, 179.

EIN S.H. & STEPHEN C.A. (1971) Intussusception. *J. Pediat. Surgery*, 6, 16.

HENDREN W.H., GREEP J.M. & PATTON A.S. (1965) Pancreatitis in childhood. *Arch. Dis. Childh.*, 40, 132.

HOLGERSEN L.O. & STANLEY-BROWN E.G. (1971) Acute appendicitis with perforation. *Am. J. Dis. Child.*, 122, 288.

JACKSON R.H. (1963) Parents, family doctors and acute appendicitis in childhood. *Brit. med. J.*, 2, 277.

JONES P.G. (1970) *Clinical Paediatric Surgery*. Bristol, John Wright.

KOPEL F.B., KIM I.C. & BARBERO G.J. (1967) Comparison of restosigmoid motility in normal children, children with recurrent abdominal pain, and children with ulcerative colitis. *Pediatrics*, 39, 539.

NAEF J. (1961) Testicular torsion in childhood. Experience with 60 cases. *Helvet. Chir. Acta*, 28, 632.

RAVITCH M.M. (1952) Consideration of errors in the diagnosis of intussusception. *Am. J. Dis. Child.*, 84, 17.

RIEMENSCHNEIDER T.A., WILSON J.F. & VERNIER R.L. (1968) Glucocorticoid induced pancreatitis in children. *Pediatrics*, 41, 428.

Silverman F.N. (1967) Regional enteritis in children. *Lancet,* 1, 207.
Williams H. (1947) Appendicitis in the young child. *Brit. med. J.,* 2, 730.
Zachary R.B. (1965) Diagnosis of the acute abdomen in childhood. *Brit. med. J.,* 1, 635.

Abdominal distension

Many toddlers are thought to have a 'big abdomen' when they are normal. If a child has some degree of lordosis, the abdomen may look as if it is distended when it is not. One occasionally sees marked distension as a result of gross constipation (causing megacolon) without Hirschsprung's disease. A fat child may have a large abdomen. In the newborn baby important causes of abdominal distension are intestinal obstruction, perforation of the alimentary, biliary or urinary tract, meconium ileus or peritonitis, tumours and Hirschsprung's disease.

Alimentary tract
   Air swallowing with a feed in infancy, or otherwise in older children
   Crying (in an infant)
   Chloramphenicol (grey syndrome in the newborn)
   Gastric dilatation, including postoperative distension
   Perforation of stomach—newborn; colon (Hirschsprung's disease); rectum (thermometer)
   Constipation, including Hirschsprung's disease
   Intestinal obstruction, including meconium ileus, annular pancreas
   Intestinal duplication; duplication cysts
   Coeliac syndrome: steatorrhoea
   Carbohydrate intolerance
Omentum and mesentery
   Cysts
   Mesenteric thrombosis

Peritoneum
  Peritonitis, malignant disease

Ascites
  Kidney—nephritis, nephrotic syndrome
  Heart—congestive heart failure
  Pericardium—constrictive pericarditis
  Liver—cirrhosis. Portal hypertension. Thombosis of portal or
      hepatic veins
  Inferior vena cava—obstruction (e.g. by Hodgkin's nodes)
  Nutritional oedema (starvation)
  Peritonitis: malignant disease: meconium peritonitis
  Lymphatic ducts—chylous ascites
    Congenital
    Acquired—trauma, obstruction of thoracic duct by tuberculous
        lymph nodes, Hodgkin's disease

Liver
  Hepatoblastoma. Cyst. Glycogen storage disease
  Mucopolysaccharidosis
  Choledochal cyst: perforation of bile duct.

Kidney
  Ectopic. Wilms's tumour. Hydronephrosis. Polycystic kidney

Adrenal
  Neuroblastoma

Spleen
  Leukaemia

Bladder
  Urethral obstruction, with perforation of urinary tract

Ovary
  Cyst

Vagina
  Hydrocolpos, haematocolpos

Uterus
  Pregnancy
  Chloramphenicol in an overdose for a newborn infant causes

abdominal distension, cyanosis, shock and other manifestations of the 'grey syndrome'.

Infants swallow large quantities of air when *crying* for a prolonged period, and the abdomen may undergo considerable distension. All infants swallow some air during feeds. Breast-fed infants swallow air excessively if they suck on an empty breast or suck too long. Bottle fed babies swallow an excess of air if the feed takes too long because the hole in the teat is too small or if they suck on a flat teat, there being a vacuum in the bottle.

Rupture of the stomach of the newborn baby leads to abdominal distension, respiratory distress, vomiting and melaena, commonly on about the third day. On auscultation no bowel sounds can be heard. *Perforation of the colon* of a newborn baby suggests Hirschsprung's disease or meconium peritonitis. Colonic perforation may follow an exchange transfusion. Four to 15 hours after the transfusion the child becomes poorly, develops abdominal distension and vomits, and there is usually blood in the stool. On auscultation no bowel sounds are heard.

Perforation of the rectum by a rectal thermometer is a well-known hazard.

Intestinal duplication or duplication cysts may cause considerable swelling of the abdomen. The cysts are often mobile and may reach a considerable size.

Constrictive pericarditis is rare in children. It follows pericarditis of unknown cause, or tuberculous or other pyogenic pericarditis.

The causes of *chylous ascites* have been listed. The diagnosis is made by aspiration of the ascitic fluid.

When there is *urethral obstruction* (due to urethral valves, etc.) there may be gross enlargement of the bladder. The diagnosis, suspected on account of the fact that the swelling involves the lower abdomen more than the upper part, is confirmed by observation of the stream of urine. In the newborn baby, perforation of the urinary tract may occur.

Finally—the possibility of *pregnancy* must not be forgotten if a girl has reached puberty.

References

Corkery J.J., Dubowitz V., Moosa A., Lister J. (1968) Colonic perforation after exchange transfusion. *Brit. med. J.*, **4**, 345.

Gwinn J.L., Lee F.A. (1970) Rupture of the stomach in the newborn infant. *Am. J. Dis. Child.*, **119**, 257.

Orme L'E.R., Eades S.M. (1968) Perforation of the bowel in the newborn as a complication of exchange transfusion. *Brit. med. J.*, **4**, 349.

Wolfson J.J. (1966) Rectal perforation in infants by thermometer. *Am. J. Dis. Child.*, **111**, 197.

Jaundice

Jaundice in infancy

The following statements can be made with little fear of contradiction:

(1) The diagnosis of the cause of jaundice in a young infant is commonly one of great difficulty.

(2) Jaundice on the first day of life must be considered to be due to haemolytic disease until proved otherwise.

(3) Physiological jaundice is not seen in the first 24 hours. With rare exceptions, jaundice after the first week in a full-term baby is not physiological and must be investigated.

(4) In physiological jaundice the urine and stools are a normal colour. There is no bilirubin in the urine and the stools contain normal bile pigments.

(5) Pale-coloured stools with a dark urine containing bilirubin signify an obstructive element. The commonest cause is neonatal hepatitis. Laboratory tests cannot at present distinguish this from congenital obliteration of the bile ducts.

(6) In the newborn period, infection is an important cause of jaundice (e.g. septicaemia), particularly when the jaundice begins after the fourth day.

(7) It is essential that every effort should be made to establish the correct diagnosis because some of the conditions demand urgent treatment.

The diagnosis

At the risk of some oversimplification, one can state that there are four main groups of causes of jaundice in the infant and young child. More than one of these causes may be operative at the same time. They are as follows:

(1) *Deficiency of the enzyme glucuronyl transferase.* Bilirubin is fat soluble, and before it can be excreted by the liver into bile or excreted in the urine, it must be converted into a water soluble form by conjugation with glucuronic acid. In the absence of glucuronyl transferase this indirectly reacting pigment ('unconjugated') accumulates in the plasma and damages the nervous system.

The following are the conditions in which deficiency of the enzyme glucuronyl transferase plays a part:

Physiological jaundice

The jaundice of prematurity

Jaundice following severe anoxia

Cretinism

Rare
  Drugs given to the mother or newborn
    Corticosteroids
    Novobiocin
  Breast milk jaundice
  Infants of diabetic mothers
  Crigler-Najjar syndrome
  Gilbert's syndrome
  Congenital pyloric stenosis
  Galactosaemia
  Adrenocortical hyperplasia

Physiological jaundice is due to a combination of immaturity of the liver with consequent transferase deficiency, and the breakdown of red cells immediately after birth. The jaundice of prematurity, whose basis is the same, is more severe than that of the newborn baby, because of greater immaturity of the enzyme system. Severe anoxia during delivery or cold injury after delivery tends to increase the jaundice.

Physiological jaundice is not seen in the first 24 hours. In a full-term baby it begins at the end of the second day and lasts for two or three days. It rarely lasts into the second week. If jaundice lasts into the second week in a full-term baby, the cause should be sought elsewhere.

The jaundice of a premature baby begins later, is more severe and lasts longer. One would not expect physiological jaundice in a premature baby in the first 48 hours. Physiological jaundice reaches its maximum about the fifth or sixth day (depending on the degree of immaturity), and in the smallest ones may last up to the 18th day. When food is withheld for 48 to 72 hours after birth, the jaundice is increased. It is reduced by early feeding.

Physiological jaundice is sometimes prolonged in a cretin because of deficiency of the transferase enzyme. This relationship between prolonged physiological jaundice and cretinism should not be forgotten.

It is thought that *corticosteriods* given to the mother during pregnancy may increase the depth of jaundice in the baby by inhibition of the transferase system. Novobiocin given to the mother or baby may act in the same way. It has recently been discovered that some babies remain jaundiced when fully *breast fed*, but that the jaundice clears as soon as they are artificially fed, returning if they are again put to the breast. It is now known that this is due to a steroid in the milk of some mothers, an isomer of pregnandiol.

The *Crigler-Najjar syndrome* is a rare recessive condition in which there is a deficiency of transferase. Extrapyramidal rigidity develops in a few weeks and persists. The picture is similar to that of kernicterus. There is no evidence of haemolysis or of obstruction.

Gilbert's disease is a much less serious congenital disease due to deficiency of the same enzyme. Mild jaundice with lassitude persists throughout life.

Occasionally infants with *congenital pyloric stenosis* have protracted jaundice with a raised serum bilirubin of indirect type (Nakai & Margaretten, 1962). The explanation of this is unknown.

The jaundice of *galactosaemia* may be due to delayed development of transferase or a toxic damage to the liver cells. When milk is given, the child goes off his food, vomits, loses weight, becomes jaundiced, and his liver and spleen enlarge.

Jaundice is sometimes an early feature of *adrenocortical hyperplasia* and of *fructose intolerance*.

It will be noted that in none of the above conditions is there bile in the urine, and in all of them the stools are of normal colour. In none of them is there haemolysis. The serum bilirubin is of the indirect or unconjugated variety.

(2) *Increased bilirubin production—mainly due to haemolysis.* The main conditions are as follows:

Congenital haemolytic disease (Rhesus or ABO incompatibility: more rarely Kell, Kidd, or Duffy group)

Hereditary spherocytosis or acholuric jaundice. Thalassaemia. Sickle cell anaemia

Drugs—Vitamin K, neomycin, camphor

Infections—septicaemia, syphilis, Weil's disease

Absorption of blood from a large cephalhaematoma or other haemorrhage

Glucose 6 phosphate dehydrogenase deficiency (p. 48)

Rarely pyruvate kinase deficiency

Jaundice on the first day must be regarded as *haemolytic disease*, due to blood group incompatibility, until proved otherwise. It is essential that a child with jaundice on the first day should be referred immediately to hospital for investigation and treatment, which may well consist of a replacement transfusion. Failure to do so without delay may lead to the death of the child or to kernicterus which is either lethal or crippling for life.

Though haemolytic disease due to rhesus incompatibility does not occur in the first pregnancy unless there has been a previous incompatible transfusion, that due to ABO incompatibility may occur in the first pregnancy, and it cannot be anticipated by tests during pregnancy. In this case the mother is usually Group O and the baby Group A, but the baby may be Group B. Rarely the mother is Group A and the infant Group B, or vice versa. The Coombs test in the infant with ABO incompatibility is commonly negative.

The diagnosis of *congenital spherocytosis* or *acholuric jaundice* is readily established by the family history of that complaint, together with examination of the child's blood for spherocytes, reticulo-cytosis and abnormal red cell fragility.

Vitamin K in an overdose increases the level of jaundice by three possible mechanisms—haemolysis, a toxic action on the liver or by competing for conjugating enzymes. It should be remembered that if the mother is given large doses of vitamin K during delivery it is likely to affect the baby.

If nappies have been stored in *camphor balls*, the baby may absorb the camphor and develop haemolytic anaemia. Neomycin may cause some degree of haemolysis.

Infections cause jaundice partly by haemolysis and partly by a toxic action on the liver which may interfere with the transferase system. The serum bilirubin is mostly unconjugated (indirect) but partly conjugated (direct). Jaundice appearing after the fourth day in a full-term infant should always be considered as infective in origin until proved otherwise. The relevant infections include septicaemia and syphilis. Sometimes the jaundice is the only manifestation of a urinary tract or other bacterial infection. The diagnosis of septicaemia would be strongly suggested by a moist umbilicus and would be confirmed by blood culture. The diagnosis of syphilis would be suspected if there were a history of inadequately treated syphilis in the mother with stigmata in the child. It would be confirmed by serological examination, remembering that in a newborn infant a false negative Wassermann reaction may be obtained for 4 to 12 weeks, and that a false positive may be found for a similar period. If the titre of the baby's blood is higher than that of the mother, or if the titre is rising, treatment should be instituted.

If a *cephalhaematoma* is a large one, the absorption of blood from it may lead to a rise in the serum bilirubin.

(3) *Interference with protein binding.* Sulphonamides and caffein sodium benzoate may increase the jaundice of a newborn baby by competing with bilirubin for protein binding and displacing bilirubin into the tissues. Kernicterus may develop with a relatively low serum bilirubin. These drugs should therefore be avoided.

(4) *Obstructive jaundice.* The following are the main causes in the newborn infant:

Neonatal hepatitis

Biliary atresia

Hepatitis due to toxoplasmosis, cytomegalovirus, herpes, syphilis

Inspissated bile

Choledochal cyst (rare). Gallstones (rare)

Dubin Johnson syndrome (rare)

Alpha$_1$ antitrypsin deficiency (pp. 143, 156)

Neonatal hepatitis is a somewhat mysterious condition of uncertain aetiology. It has occurred in two or three children of the same family. In some, the rubella virus has been isolated (Stern & Williams, 1966). It may be the end result of several conditions such as serum hepatitis in the mother. The relationship of neonatal hepatitis to biliary atresia is uncertain. Jaundice due to neonatal hepatitis may be present at birth or appear during the first week or two. It is of varying duration and may last for several months before clearing.

There are no certain means of distinguishing neonatal hepatitis from *biliary atresia*. An American paper on neonatal jaundice described 73 liver function tests recommended for this age period. In general the serum glutamic oxaloacetic transaminase (SGOT) is higher in hepatitis than in atresia, but this cannot be relied upon. Even a liver biopsy may not provide a definite answer. It is important, however, to determine whether there is any obstructive lesion of the biliary tract which can be corrected by surgery: only a very small number of cases can be corrected, but one must give the child the benefit of the doubt. This can be determined by limited laparotomy with a cholangiogram after injecting dye into the gall bladder and biopsy of a specimen of liver. If nothing is or can be done for an infant with biliary atresia, he continues to have severe jaundice with biliary cirrhosis and dies in a few months, or rarely a few years.

Hepatitis due to *toxoplasmosis* or *cytomegalovirus* is rare. The diagnosis is made by serological methods.

Obstructive jaundice may occasionally develop in infants suffering from haemolytic anaemia due to *blood group incompatibility*.

This has been ascribed to inspissated bile blocking the bile duct. It is rare, but there have been instances in which the jaundice has cleared after the duct has been washed through at laparotomy.

A choledochal cyst is a rare cause of obstructive jaundice.

The *Dubin Johnson syndrome* is a rare type of chronic jaundice with bile in the urine, due to an inability of the hepatic cells to excrete conjugated bilirubin.

Jaundice after infancy

(1) *Obstructive*

By far the commonest cause of jaundice after infancy is *infective hepatitis*. There will be bile in the urine and the stools will be clay coloured. It could also be due to serum hepatitis, if the child has had a transfusion, or has been given injections with a contaminated needle.

Toxic hepatitis can be caused by scores of *drugs* (Sherlock, 1964). These include antibiotics, such as acetazolamide, amitriptyline, amphetamine, anabolic steroids, antimetabolites, cephalexin, chloramphenicol, chloroquine, erythromycin estolate, ethionamide, ethosuccimide, gold, griseofulvin, halothane, imipramine, indomethacin, iron, isoniazid, kanamycin, lincomycin, methimazole, methotrexate, nalidixic acid, neomycin, nitrofurantoin, novobiocin, oleandomycin, oxyphenisatin (dulcolax), P.A.S., penicillin, phenacetin, pheneturide, phenothiazines, phenytoin, pyrazinamide, quinine, rifampicin, sulphonamides, testosterone, tetracycline, thiouracil, troxidone, vancomycin and vincristine. It can also be caused by a wide variety of poisons, such as phosphorus, iron, arsenic, bismuth or fungi.

Cirrhosis of the liver in its late stages causes jaundice as in adults. Biliary cirrhosis may result from fibrocystic disease of the pancreas.

Weil's disease (leptospirosis) is a rare cause of jaundice. It is characterised by jaundice, fever, leucocytosis, albuminuria and haemorrhages. It is diagnosed by agglutination tests, isolation of the spirochaete in the blood or inoculation of a guinea-pig.

Infectious mononucleosis is on rare occasions complicated by jaundice.

(2) *Haemolytic*

In jaundice due to haemolysis the urine does not contain bile and the stools are of a normal colour. The causes are congenital spherocytosis (acholuric jaundice), sickle cell anaemia and thalassaemia, and acquired (autoimmune) haemolytic anaemia. The diagnosis of haemolysis is made by the finding of reticulocytosis in the blood, raised serum bilirubin of the indirect type, excess of urobilinogen in the urine and of bile pigments in the stools. In acholuric jaundice there is in addition an enlargement of the spleen, spherocytes in the blood film and increased red cell fragility. Sickle cell anaemia is diagnosed in some cases in the ordinary blood film, but in most other cases by simple laboratory methods to demonstrate the effect of low oxygen tension on the shape of the cell.

For the haemolytic-uraemic syndrome, see p. 48.

References

ANON (1965) Bile duct perforation in infancy. *Brit. med. J.*, **1**, 174.

AREY J.B., BLANC W.A., CRAIG J.M., GELLIS S.S., HARRIS R.C., KAYE R., LANDING B.H., NEWTON W.A., SASS-KORSTAK A., STOWENS D., YAKOVAC W.C. & ZUELZER W.W. (1962) Persistent jaundice in infancy. *J. Pediat.*, **61**, 111.

ARIAS I.M., GARTNER L.M., SEIFTER S. & FURMAN M. (1964) Neonatal jaundice and breast feeding. *J. clin. Invest.*, **43**, 2037.

BROWN A.K. (1962) Neonatal jaundice. *Pediat. Clinics. N. Am.*, **9**, 575.

DANKS D.M. (1965) Prolonged neonatal obstructive jaundice. *Clin. Pediat.*, **4**, 499.

HANSHAW J.B. (1966) Congenital and acquired cytomegalovirus infection. *Pediat. Clinics. N. Am.*, **13**, 279.

NAKAI H. & MARGARETTEN W. (1962) Protracted jaundice associated with hypertrophic pyloric stenosis. *Pediatrics*, **29**, 198.

ROONEY J.C., HILL D.J. & DANKS D.M. (1971) Jaundice associated with bacterial infection in the newborn. *Am. J. Dis. Child.*, **122**, 39.

SHERLOCK S. (1964) Jaundice due to drugs. *Proc. R. Soc. Med.*, **57**, 881.

STERN H. & WILLIAMS B.M. (1966) Isolation of rubella virus in a case of neonatal giant cell hepatitis. *Lancet*, **1**, 293.

ZUELZER W.W. & BROWN A.K. (1961) Neonatal jaundice. *Am. J. Dis. Child.*, **101**, 87.

Persistent cyanosis

Peripheral cyanosis is a normal feature of normal newborn infants. The limbs are cyanosed, while the face and trunk is a normal pink. The cyanosis lasts a few days only.

Causes of *persistent generalised cyanosis* in an infant include the following:

Congenital heart disease
Severe chest disease (acute only). Respiratory distress syndrome.
   Cerebral oedema or haemorrhage
Methaemoglobinaemia
   (i) Congenital
   (ii) Absorption of aniline from laundry marks on clothes
   (iii) Other poisons—acetanilide, dinitrophenol, nitrites, phenylazopyridine, potassium perchlorate.
   (iv) Phenytoin taken by breast-feeding mother
Sulphhaemoglobinaemia

Congenital heart disease is the most common cause of persistent cyanosis in an infant. In a newborn baby, the usual causes are complete transposition of the great vessels or cor triloculare. Other causes are a truncus arteriosus or tricuspid atresia. In the first two of these there may be no cardiac murmur. After the newborn period the usual lesion is Fallot's tetralogy. It can also be due to a right to left shunt when there is a patent ductus arteriosus with coarctation of the aorta proximal to the ductus. Other causes are a hypoplastic left heart, isolated pulmonary stenosis or atresia, tricuspid atresia and a persistent truncus. The diagnosis is established by the usual investigations—x-ray of the chest for heart shape and size, ECG, cardiac catheterisation and angiocardiography. The rather non-specific condition termed *fibroelastosis* may also cause persistent cyanosis with heart failure.

Severe chest disease is an unlikely cause of persistent cyanosis in a baby, except in an acute illness such as the respiratory distress syndrome or atelectasis. A baby may rapidly develop respiratory distress, bronchitis, cyanosis and intercostal retraction after the accidental *inhalation of talcum powder*.

Persistent generalised cyanosis in association with dyspnoea is likely to be due to *atelectasis*, or possibly *pneumothorax, mediastinal or lobar emphysema* or a large *diaphragmatic hernia*. It must be remembered that atelectasis may itself be due to a *cerebral haemorrhage*. One must not forget to palpate the anterior fontanelle and the sutures for evidence of increased intracranial pressure.

Methaemoglobinaemia may be congenital, or it may result from the absorption of aniline from laundry marks which have been applied *after* the nappies or clothes have been boiled. If they are applied before boiling, absorption does not occur. Methaemoglobinaemia has occurred in rural areas as a result of the presence of *nitrates* in well water used for making up the feeds. A variety of other rather unlikely poisons may cause the condition. When a lactating mother takes phenytoin, the baby may be cyanosed as a result.

Babies may develop cyanosis and methaemoglobinaemia as a result of eating spinach, especially if they are also given the water in which it was boiled. It is due to nitrates in the spinach.

Cyanosis may result from polycythaemia.

Sulphhaemoglobinaemia is a rare congenital metabolic disorder.

In the older child the likely causes of persistent cyanosis are *congenital heart disease, pulmonary hypertension* or *pulmonary fibrosis*.

References

British Medical Journal, Annotation (1966) Spinach, a risk to babies. *Brit. med. J.*, **1**, 250.
British Medical Journal (1969) Accidental inhalation of talcum powder. *Brit. med. J.*, **4**, 5.
LEES M.H. (1970) Cyanosis of the newborn infant. *J. Pediat.*, **77**, 484.

Cyanotic attacks in the newborn

Everyone who looks after newborn babies is conversant with cyanotic attacks ('apnoeic attacks'), but the subject is inadequately discussed in most textbooks. A baby, usually in his first few days, but sometimes a little later, is found to be ashen grey in colour and not breathing. The condition is far more common in the premature baby than in the full-term one, and the smaller the premature baby the more common are cyanotic attacks. These attacks are particularly common during feeds because of milk entering the trachea.

The causes of cyanotic attacks may be grouped as follows:

Depression of the respiratory centre
    Prematurity
    Cerebral oedema or haemorrhage
    Brain defects
    Meningitis
    Respiratory distress syndrome

Obstruction of the airway
    Vomited material inhaled
    Milk entering the trachea
    Thick mucus, etc.
    Nasal obstruction, including choanal atresia

Convulsions
    Hypocalcaemia (tetany)
    Hypoglycaemia
    Hypernatraemia
    Tetanus
    Infections
    Cerebral oedema, haemorrhages, defects
Primary alveolar hypoventilation (rare)

In a study in Sheffield, we found that congenital heart disease was a rare cause of cyanotic attacks.

Depression or immaturity of the respiratory centre is an important cause of cyanotic attacks. It may be due to analgesic or anaesthetic drugs administered to the mother during labour. In the case of prematurity, phasic respiration, including Cheyne-Stokes breathing, is a normal finding in small premature infants; some cyanotic attacks are due to failure to restart breathing after the normal brief apnoeic phase. Any sort of stimulation, such as pinching the toe, causes the baby to breathe again. In premature or full-term infants, cerebral oedema, subdural or cerebral haemorrhage or serious congenital brain defects may cause apnoeic attacks. When a one or two week old baby who has been previously well develops cyanotic attacks, pyogenic meningitis must be remembered as a possible cause. It has been suggested that there may be a connection between apnoeic attacks and a rise of temperature in the incubator (Sinclair 1970).

Obstruction of the airway is a major cause of apnoeic attacks. The treatment must include aspiration to ensure that the airway is patent. Nasal obstruction may cause apnoeic attacks because the newborn baby does not usually open his mouth to breathe when the nose is blocked. Choanal atresia is rare but of the utmost importance, in that the correct treatment is easy to apply and life-saving. It is due to a web or membrane behind the palate. If it is complete, the child gasps for breath or has apnoeic attacks, but his distress is immediately relieved by crying or by the insertion of an oral airway pending elective surgery. Cyanosis may be due to obstruction of the airway by a vascular ring.

Many cyanotic attacks are *convulsions*. The newborn infant does not have major convulsions. He may twitch and he may have apnoeic attacks. Convulsions are an important and frequent cause of cyanotic attacks. The causes of neonatal convulsions have been discussed on p. 186. In that section the importance of diagnosing and therefore treating one of the main causes of convulsions in the newborn, namely hypoglycaemia, is emphasised. Cyanotic attacks may be due to primary alveolar hypoventilation ('Ondine's curse'), in which there is shallow breathing, often with apnoeic attacks, with chronic respiratory acidosis—probably due to failure of the central mechanism of respiration.

Cyanotic attacks must not be taken lightly. They carry a high mortality. Some of the causes are readily treatable and it is important that the cause should be determined.

References

GAIRDNER D. (1965) Respiratory distress in the newborn in *Recent Advances in Paediatrics*. London, Churchill.

HOBOLTH N., BUCHMAN G. & SANDBERG L.E. (1967) Congenital choanal atresia. *Acta Paediat. Scand.*, **56**, 286.

ILLINGWORTH R.S. (1957) Cyanotic attacks in newborn infants. *Arch. Dis. Childh.*, **32**, 328.

SCHAFFER A.J. & AVERY M.E. (1971) *Diseases of the Newborn*. Philadelphia, Saunders.

SINCLAIR J.S. (1970) The premature baby who forgets to breathe. *New Engl. J. Med.*, 282, 508.

Dyspnoea in the newborn

The following conditions should be considered:

Respiratory distress syndrome (hyaline membrane disease)
Massive aspiration of amniotic fluid
Mediastinal or lobar emphysema, pneumothorax or air cyst
Atelectasis
Cerebral anoxia or haemorrhage
Diaphragmatic hernia
Diaphragmatic paralysis
Intrauterine pneumonia
Tracheo-oesophageal fistula
Choanal atresia (p. 126)
Anaemia
Congenital heart disease: heart failure
Vascular ring
Accidental inhalation of talc

For an excellent discussion of this difficult subject, the reader is referred to the book by Schaffer.

The most common cause of dyspnoea in the newborn baby is the *respiratory distress syndrome* ('hyaline membrane syndrome'). This occurs under three main circumstances—when the baby is born prematurely, is born by Caesarian section or is born by a diabetic mother. It is more common in boys than girls. Within the first hour of birth there is a rising respiration rate. The baby begins to make a grunting sound on expiration. There is indrawing of the lower part of the chest and sternum and there may be some cyanosis or cyanotic attacks. On examination there may be râles in the chest and dullness on percussion or signs of emphysema. There may be signs of heart failure with peripheral circulatory failure, cyanosis and muffled heart sounds. The x-ray of the chest shows a characteristic picture. The condition may be confused with most of the conditions below.

Massive aspiration of amniotic fluid. This occurs particularly in post-mature babies and in babies delivered by forceps or breech, and after prolonged labour, placental insufficiency or prolapse of the cord, or a cord which has been tightly knotted or tightly round the neck. The child is apt to be shocked as a result of anoxia, and soon after birth, usually within three or four hours, he becomes dyspnoeic. There may be associated signs of brain injury, such as a high-pitched cry or an absent or exaggerated Moro reflex. There may be complicating atelectasis, emphysema, pneumothorax or pneumonia.

Mediastinal emphysema and pneumothorax are associated with dyspnoea, rapid shallow respirations and cyanosis. The chest may appear to be over-distended, and in the case of pneumothorax there will be decreased movement on one side, with displacement of the trachea and apex beat to the opposite side. In either case there will be hyperresonance over the affected area, and in the case of mediastinal emphysema there may be a characteristic crunching sound with each heart beat (Hamman's sign). A large air-containing cyst cannot be distinguished clinically from pneumothorax.

Atelectasis may be associated with persistent cyanosis and feeble respiratory movements. The apex beat is deflected towards the affected side. Agenesis of the lung causes dullness and decreased breath sounds on the affected side with gross mediastinal displacement to the same side. It can be difficult to be sure that the respiratory symptoms are not due to cerebral oedema or haemorrhage.

Diaphragmatic hernia is an acute emergency if the hernia is large. There is commonly cyanosis and dyspnoea from birth, though these may develop later. The chest may be overfilled while the abdomen may be flat. There is resonance or dullness.

Paralysis of the diaphragm is most commonly associated with Erb's Palsy. Respirations are rapid and there are decreased respiratory movements on the affected side with decreased sounds at the base.

Intrauterine pneumonia may follow prolonged rupture of the membranes. The initial symptoms are usually non-specific. The child is ill at birth, shows little inclination to suck and may vomit.

The temperature may be subnormal or raised. He has rapid and often grunting respirations but does not usually cough. The abdomen may be distended. The condition has to be distinguished from staphylococcal pneumonia which develops later. The onset is usually insidious, the child becoming ill and toxic in appearance. He may develop an empyema or pyopneumothorax.

A *tracheo-oesophageal fistula* will cause dyspnoea if the diagnosis is delayed until after feeds are given, with resultant regurgitation or entry of milk into the trachea.

Severe anaemia and *heart failure* are important though rare causes of dyspnoea, requiring immediate treatment. The symptoms of heart failure include feeding difficulties, rapid respirations and oedema. It may be caused by myocarditis, congenital heart disease, fibroelastosis, glycogen storage disease, heart block, paroxysmal tachycardia, respiratory distress syndrome and septicaemia.

A *vascular ring* may cause dyspnoea and stridor with cyanosis during feeding.

The features of the various conditions may be summarised as follows (modified from Schaffer):

Severe dyspnoea immediately after birth—suggesting a major malformation

Violent respiratory efforts with no air entry—laryngeal atresia, choanal atresia

Early dyspnoea—respiratory distress syndrome, diaphragmatic hernia, massive aspiration, intrauterine pneumonia

Sudden dyspnoea after a few hours—pneumothorax, atelectasis

Overfull chest—lobar emphysema, pneumothorax, diaphragmatic hernia

Asymmetrical chest—diaphragmatic hernia, diaphragmatic paralysis, pneumothorax, air containing cyst, lobar emphysema, pulmonary agenesis

Hyperresonance—lobar emphysema, pneumothorax, air-containing cyst

Local dullness—atelectasis, tumour, diaphragmatic hernia

Wheeze—vascular ring, unilobular emphysema, mediastinal tumour

Stridor—see p. 145.

Grunting respirations—respiratory distress syndrome, pneumonia
For the accidental inhalation of talc, see p. 124.

Reference

LEES M.H. (1969) Heart failure in the newborn infant. *J. Pediat.*, **75,** 139.

Epistaxis

Epistaxis is rare in infancy but common in later childhood.

The cause of epistaxis is by no means always obvious. It may be due to nose-picking, injury, or dilated veins in the nasal septum. Telangiectasia of the nasal septum, often accompanied by telangiectasia on the face or elsewhere, is a familial cause of epistaxis. Any foreign body may cause nose bleeds. Nose bleeding may occur with acute congestion in an upper respiratory tract infection, measles or influenza, in much the same way as bleeding occurs from the throat in the presence of acute tonsillitis.

Many blood diseases, such as haemophilia, Christmas disease, thrombocytopenic purpura and the leukaemias may cause epistaxis. Epistaxis may occur in the terminal stages of kidney or liver disease.

Severe whooping cough is not often seen now, but it used to be a common cause of nose bleeds.

Atrophic rhinitis and nasal polypi are other possible causes. Nasal diphtheria and congenital syphilis are now rarely seen, but they used to be important causes of a sero-sanguinous nasal discharge. A unilateral sanguino-purulent nasal discharge should be ascribed to a foreign body until proved otherwise.

Halitosis

It is difficult to find discussion of the causation of halitosis.

Most of the textbooks seen by me, whether general or devoted to otorhinolaryngology, make no mention of the symptom. One book devoted a page to the condition, but listed such unlikely causes as mercury, iodide, bismuth or lead poisoning, cirrhosis of the liver, nasal allergy, 'chronic gastrointestinal disorders', spicy foods, and a low fat diet. Carious teeth are mentioned as a cause, but I doubt whether this is common. The symptom may arise from food debris between teeth which are too close together for proper cleaning to be possible. Halitosis in an ill child may be due to acute tonsillitis, diphtheria or Vincent's infection, bronchiectasis or lung abscess. Severe halitosis of recent origin, especially if there is a nasal discharge, would suggest a foreign body in the nose. The symptom may be due to the child eating onions or garlic.

Atrophic rhinitis occurs predominantly at puberty or later, but may begin in early infancy. It is almost confined to girls. It often starts after some illness. In adolescence it is worse at the time of menstruation. The nasal cavity becomes greatly widened and the halitosis is extreme. It is often a familiar feature.

I consider that it is true to say that if atrophic rhinitis and a foreign body in the nose have been eliminated, it is unlikely that one will find the cause of halitosis in an otherwise well child.

References

Drug and Therapeutics Bulletin (1969) Halitosis. **7**, 79.
TAYLOR M. & YOUNG A. (1961) Histopathological and histochemical studies on atrophic rhinitis. *J. Laryngology and Otology*, **75**, 574.

Stomatitis and gingivitis

Stomatitis may be due to the following causes:

Infection
Allergy
Avitaminosis
The effect of drugs
The Stevens Johnson syndrome

Infections causing stomatitis include herpes, Vincent's infection, the Coxsackie virus and monilia. It is probable that other viruses may cause it. Herpes causes vesicles on the tongue without necrosis, while Vincent's organisms cause necrotic ulcers on the tips of papillae and involves the gums and tonsils. Vincent's infection is confirmed by the smell and by a smear for the spirochaetes. Coxsackie stomatitis closely resembles herpes, with small vesicles on the tongue and mucous membranes, but with more tendency to lymph node involvement. Thrush infection resembles curds of milk on the tongue and buccal mucosa, but the white patches cannot be removed by a swab. *Allergic aphthae* are indistinguishable from those of herpes.

Stomatitis may be caused by *avitaminosis*, especially ariboflavinosis and other deficiencies of the Vitamin B complex, particularly in children on synthetic diets without adequate vitamin supplements. Scurvy may also cause it.

Drugs which cause stomatitis include actimomycin D, ethosuccimide, gold, meprobamate, 6 mercaptopurine, methotrexate, troxidone and vincristine.

The Stevens Johnson syndrome is more common in boys than girls. There is a severe stomatitis, with erythematous papular lesions, vesicles or bullae beginning on the extensor surfaces of the extremities, and spreading to the trunk, neck and scalp. There may be lesions on the conjunctivae, nares, anorectal junction, vulva and urethral meatus. The child is poorly and feverish, and may have kidney, joint or pulmonary involvement. The cause is not always known, but it may be due to anticonvulsants (barbiturates, carbamazepine, troxidone), aspirin, penicillin, quinine or sulphonamides.

Gingivitis may be due to the following causes:

Infection
Drugs
Avitaminoses
Dental caries
Overcrowding of teeth
Malocclusion
Mouthbreathing
Familial type

The gums in gingivitis are red, boggy and bleed easily.

Infections which cause it include herpes, Vincent's infection thrush, streptococcal and staphylococcal organisms. Herpes zoster or herpes simplex may cause vesicles on the gums with underlying inflammation. Vincent's infection and thrush have already been described. Staphylococcal gingivitis is usually found in children severely ill from another cause. The gums in streptococcal gingivitis are characteristically bright red and the child is ill. In both these cases the diagnosis is made by culture.

The principal *drug* which causes gingivitis is phenytoin. The gingivitis subsides within three to six months after discontinuing the drug. It is not related to the blood phenytoin level.

Avitaminoses, especially scurvy, cause the gums to be inflamed and liable to bleed.

Dental decay and *stagnating food between teeth*, often associated with overcrowding of teeth, are causes. *Malocclusion* is often related.

Mouthbreathing causes gingivitis, but the gum trouble is more often due to a short upper lip providing an inadequate lip seal and so drying the gingivae.

There is a rare familial type of *fibromatous gingivitis*, resembling the gingivitis caused by phenytoin.

Dryness in the mouth

This may be due to *dehydration*, or to a variety of *drugs*, including amitriptyline, amphetamine, antihistamines, atropine, codeine, cyclopentolate, hyoscine, imipramine, the phenothiazine group and vitamin A overdosage. Cyclopentolate drops may cause an acute toxic psychosis, a dry mouth, ataxia and delirium. It may occasionally be due to mouthbreathing.

Reference

ADCOCK E.W. (1971) Cyclopentolate (Cyclogyl) toxicity in pediatric patients. *J. Pediat.*, **79,** 127.

Toothgrinding

Toothgrinding in sleep may occur in a normal child, but tooth-grinding in a child who is awake is usually an indication of mental subnormality.

It is said to be an occasional side effect of fenfluramine.

Salivation and drooling

Conditions to consider include the following:

Normal variation

Eruption of a tooth

Mental subnormality

Abnormality of nervous control—cerebral palsy, motor neurone disease, facial palsy, polyneuritis, myasthenia, myotonia dystrophica

Stomatitis

Drugs and poisons

Oesophageal atresia

Perforation of the pharynx

Familial dysautonomia

Most normal babies lack control of the flow of saliva until 12 months or so of age. Some seem to have more saliva than others, and their clothes are constantly wet. Salivation is a common sign of teething. Drooling sometimes continues for years without apparent reason. It is sometimes associated with mouth breathing. Mentally defective children, being late in all aspects of development, except occasionally sitting and walking, are late in controlling the saliva, and this may be one of the troublesome features of mental deficiency from the mother's point of view. Children with cerebral palsy, especially of the athetoid type, are particularly liable to 'drool' for several years, partly, perhaps, because of incoordination of the tongue and lips.

It seems likely that drooling is more often due to failure to swallow or retain saliva than to excessive salivation (Smith and Goode, 1970). This difficulty may be due to a variety of conditions such as cerebral palsy, facial palsy, myasthenia, myotonia dystrophia, or stricture of the oesophagus.

Drooling may be associated with excessive salivation caused by stomatitis, iodides or mercury poisoning. Salivation is a feature of poisoning by organophosphorus insecticides and by the anti-cholinesterase eye drops phospholine iodide. Nitrazepam used in the treatment of epilepsy may cause excessive salivation and lachrymation. Ethionamide may cause salivation. Salivation may be a feature in the newborn baby borne by a heroin addict.

Salivation is a feature of oesophageal atresia or perforation of the pharynx (p. 63).

References

FREEDMAN A.R. (1966) Familial dysautonomia. *Clinical Pediatrics*, **5**, 265.
SMITH R.A. & GOODE R.L. (1970) Sialorrhoea. *New Engl. J. Med.*, **283**, 917.

Difficulty in sucking and swallowing

The diagnosis of the cause of sucking and swallowing problems in infancy is liable to be a matter of great difficulty. I have reviewed the subject fully elsewhere (1969). I suggested the following classification:

(1) Gross congenital anatomical defects
        Palate—cleft
        Tongue—macroglossia, cysts, tumours
        Retronasal space—choanal atresia
        Mandible—micrognathia
        Temperomandibular joint—ankylosis, hypoplasia
        Pharynx—cyst, diverticulum
        Oesophagus—atresia, fistula, stenosis, web
        Thorax—vascular ring

(2) Neuromuscular defects

Delayed maturation—normal variation, prematurity, mental subnormality

Cerebral palsy

Cranial nerve nuclei or tracts

Bulbar or suprabulbar palsy

Möbius syndrome—congenital facial diplegia

Congenital laryngeal stridor

Chalasia or achalasia of the oesophagus

Muscular dystrophy, myotonic dystrophy, myasthenia gravis, hypotonias

Syndromes—Cornelia de Lange, Riley, Prader Willi

Rumination, tongue thrusting

(3) Acute infections

Stomatitis

Oesophagitis

Poliomyelitis

Diphtheria

Tetanus

Space will not permit a full discussion of all these numerous conditions, and I propose to mention a few only. Even an expert is liable to find the establishment of the diagnosis a matter of considerable complexity.

For the most part the group consisting of gross congenital anatomical defects is not difficult to diagnose. Choanal atresia is discussed on p. 126.

The differential diagnosis of the large group of neuromuscular defects is much more difficult. An important cause is delayed maturation. This may occur in normal full term infants, the problem resolving itself in a week or two or sometimes much longer; it is usual in the small premature baby, and common in the mentally subnormal child, who is characteristically late in all aspects of development. The child with cerebral palsy is liable to have difficulty in sucking and swallowing because of stiffness and incoordination of the relevant muscles. The early signs of the spastic form include delayed motor development (e.g., poor head control), a small head circumference, excessive muscle tone and exaggerated tendon jerks. I have discussed the early diagnosis in detail elsewhere (1970).

Bulbar and suprabulbar palsy are important causes of dysphagia. There may be paresis of the palate and other cranial nerve palsies, often with jaw clonus and a jaw jerk.

Myasthenia, the hypotonias, the Riley and Prader Willi syndrome and rumination are discussed elsewhere in this book. For neonatal tetanus see p. 189.

References

ILLINGWORTH R.S. (1969) Sucking and swallowing difficulties in infancy. Diagnostic problems of dysphagia. *Arch. Dis. Childh.*, **44,** 655.
ILLINGWORTH R.S. (1972) *Development of the Infant and Young Child: Normal and Abnormal.* Edinburgh, Churchill Livingstone.

Delayed dentition and missing teeth

Delayed dentition is common in normal children. There are wide variations in the age at which the first tooth appears. Some babies are born with a tooth or teeth, while others may not cut the first tooth until after the first birthday.

The following are causes of abnormal delay in dentition and of teeth being missing:

Supernumerary teeth, particularly upper central and lateral incisors, impeding the eruption of the permanent ones.

Overlong retention of deciduous teeth, for unknown reasons.

Crowding of the jaw—as a result of the teeth being unduly large or the jaw being unduly small. These are often familiar features.

Cretinism.

Premature loss of deciduous teeth. This may be due to decay or rarely to hypophosphatasia (in which there may be rickets, with a low plasma phosphatase).

Missing teeth, apart from the usual loss of teeth, may be due to *ectodermal dysplasia.* There may be missing upper lateral incisors, lower third molars or premolars. The condition affects predominantly the permanent teeth and is familial. There are likely to be other signs of the disease—a dry skin, sparse hair and abnormal nails.

There is a rare form of familial *anodontia*.

Colds and nasal discharge

The term *snuffles* refers to a clear mucoid nasal discharge sometimes seen in babies in their first few weeks. The reason for the discharge is uncertain. On microscopy there is no excess of polymorphonuclear white cells, such as would suggest infection, and no excess of eosinophils, such as would suggest allergy. The baby blows bubbles as he breaths and may have some difficulty in feeding because of blockage of the nose. It cures itself in a few weeks.

Even the youngest babies may develop a *cold*, and the common complications such as otitis media may result. Other complications include laryngitis and bronchopneumonia. The baby may have difficulty in breathing because he does not open his mouth when the nose is obstructed. He may fail to gain weight or actually lose weight. Some babies develop diarrhoea when they have a cold. An ordinary respiratory infection in an infant or young child may lead to alarming dehydration requiring hospital treatment. Two of the most troublesome complications of colds in the young child are a postnasal discharge and asthmatic bronchitis (p. 144). Culture of the nasal discharge in a baby suffering from a cold not infrequently yields haemolytic streptococci.

Many mistake the normal *sneezing* of the newborn baby for a cold. Babies in their first few weeks sneeze frequently without any evidence of infection.

Allergic rhinitis is commonly mistaken for colds in older infants and children. The persistence of the nasal discharge, the fact that it is clear and mucoid, together with the continual sneezing, should alert one to the true diagnosis. If the child is never free from a nasal discharge, if the child's nose is running when there has been no history of exposure to infection, or if there is a strong family history of allergy, one would suspect allergic rhinitis rather than coryza. The presence of a wheeze would certainly suggest allergy, though the difficulty of a cold precipitating an attack of asthmatic bronchitis is discussed on p. 144. When in doubt, a nasal smear should be examined under the microscope: if the proportion of eosinophils exceeds three per cent, one would think that allergic rhinitis is likely.

When a child has purulent nasal discharge between colds, he must be presumed to have an *antrum infection*. This can occur even in infancy. In making this diagnosis, which is confirmed by direct inspection of the nares and by x-ray of the antrum, one must distinguish the usual muco-purulent discharge at the end of a cold. An antrum infection is a fairly common complication of fibrocystic disease of the pancreas.

A unilateral purulent nasal discharge suggests a *foreign body* in the nose. When diphtheria was prevalent, a serosanguineous unilateral discharge suggested *nasal diphtheria*.

A persistent nasal discharge is an early feature of Riley's syndrome (p. 40). Certain *drugs* may be responsible for nasal congestion or discharge. They include reserpine given to the mother during pregnancy, causing nasal congestion in the neonate; trimeprazine given later in childhood, and iodides.

Cough

Acute cough

The important conditions to consider include the following:

Acute respiratory infections
   Colds and their complications
   Pneumonia
   Asthma and asthmatic bronchitis
Measles
Whooping cough
Foreign body in the bronchus

Chronic cough

Habit or tic
Smoking
Postnasal discharge
    The sequela of a cold
    Adenoids
    Antrum infection
Whooping cough
Bronchitis and asthma
Fibrocystic disease of the pancreas
Partial collapse of the lung
Small tracheo-oesophageal fistula (in an infant)
Overspill from chalasia of the oesophagus or hiatus hernia
Bronchiectasis
Foreign body in the bronchus
Tuberculosis
Allergy
Congenital heart disease
Immunological deficiency

Acute cough

Cough is an unusual symptom in the newborn. There is usually
little or no cough when the infant has the respiratory distress syndrome, atelectasis or pneumonia. Cough with choking in a newborn infant may be due to a tracheoesophageal fistula or oesophageal
atresia, congenital laryngeal cleft or perforation of the pharynx.
After the newborn period, the principal cause of cough is a respiratory infection. A cold may be followed by laryngitis, tracheitis,
bronchitis or pneumonia. In some children, colds are followed by
asthmatic bronchitis (p. 144), or true asthma. An acute attack of
cough with dyspnoea may be due to the accidental inhalation of
talc.

A pneumonia-like illness may occur in *sickle cell disease*.

An acute respiratory infection may be the initial sign of *measles*.
In this case Koplik's spots will be found in the buccal mucosa.

Cough is *not* due to teething, and one cannot visualise any mechanism whereby the eruption of a tooth through the periosteum would cause a cough. Neither is cough due to an 'enlarged thymus'.

An infant may have no immunity from *whooping cough* at birth, and may therefore develop the infection from the newborn period onwards. A cough which is worse at night and which repeatedly makes the child sick should be regarded as whooping cough until proved otherwise. The typical whoop may not be heard at all if the attack is a mild one or has been modified by partial immunisation (e.g. in a two or three year old, who was immunised in the first six months and did not receive a booster dose a year later). The whoop may not be heard in a young infant. In any case the whoop may not be heard for a week or two after the onset. The whoop is not specific for pertussis. A whoop may be heard in another condition in which there is inspissated mucus which the child has difficulty in bringing up—namely *fibrocystic disease of the pancreas.*

In an uncomplicated whooping cough there are no abnormal physical signs on auscultation, but there will be signs if there is a serious complication such as bronchopneumonia or extensive collapse of the lung.

The diagnosis of whooping cough is confirmed by culture of a fresh pernasal swab (not postnasal). The diagnosis can be presumed if the child who has typical symptoms also has a lymphocytosis. Not all children with whooping cough show this blood change, but two thirds do in the first two weeks of the infection, 85 per cent in the third week and half show it in the fourth week. Lymphocytosis is less likely in the first six months.

Connor (1970) described a whooping cough-like illness due to an adenovirus 12 infection. A similar illness may be due to the cytomegalovirus.

The possibility of a *foreign body* in the bronchus must never be forgotten, especially when there is a history of the sudden onset of a severe cough. This may be followed by a silent period and then by fever, cough and signs of infection in the obstructed lung. There may be a history of a child eating peanuts or playing with small objects which could have been inhaled. Whenever a child presents with a cough of sudden onset, without a preceding cold, or with collapse of a lobe of the lung, the diagnosis of a foreign body in the bronchus must be eliminated. In a review of 230 cases of inhaled foreign bodies, 46·5 per cent of all foreign bodies were nuts (Pyman, 1971). There is often a delay in the onset of signs and symptoms. One hundred and six of the children presented only with a wheeze without a cough.

Chronic cough

A cough may be due to a *habit, tic,* or *attention seeking device.* A common and troublesome cause of cough in a young child is a *postnasal discharge.* The usual cause of this is a cold. The child has little or no cough when up and about, but coughs continually as soon as he lies down. The postnasal discharge can be seen on inspection of the throat. The child may be helped by sleeping in the prone position.

Adenoids or antrum infection may cause a cough by the same mechanism. If a child has a postnasal obstruction and a postnasal discharge, with nasal speech and recurrent otitis media, the likely diagnosis is adenoids. If the ear, nose and throat specialist is unable to obtain a good view of the postnasal space in a young child, a lateral x-ray of the nasopharynx will show a pad of adenoids.

If there is a chronic antrum infection there will almost certainly be a history of a persistent purulent nasal discharge between colds, or of a postnasal discharge with cough. There may be an allergic basis. The diagnosis is confirmed by an x-ray.

Following *whooping cough*, a cough may persist for some weeks or months, and may recur. It is always as well to have an x-ray taken in case there is a partial collapse of a lung.

Fibrocystic disease of the pancreas is discussed on p. 10. The diagnosis should be suspected when a child has a persistent or frequently recurring cough with pulmonary infections, except when the cough immediately follows an ordinary cold.

When a child has an acute respiratory infection and fails to make the usual recovery, feeling tired and off colour, the cough continuing, one suspects a *partial collapse of the lung.* There may be râles localised to one base, or even bronchovesicular breathing. Sometimes there are no definite signs, but the x-ray photograph establishes the diagnosis.

When a young infant regularly coughs during feeds, the possibility of a *small tracheo-oesophageal fistula* has to be considered. The diagnosis would be established by a lipiodol swallow. A lateral film of the chest may show distension of the oesophagus by air.

When an infant regurgitates a great deal and also has a cough, the cause could be *chalasia of the oesophagus or hiatus hernia*, with inhalation of some regurgitated material into the lung. The diagnosis would be established by a barium swallow.

Bronchiectasis is now rarely seen in British children. It would be suspected if the child had a persistent productive cough with clubbing of the fingers and an antrum infection. It may be due to an underlying congenital abnormality. The diagnosis would be established by an x-ray and bronchogram.

A chronic cough following an acute onset could be due to a *foreign body* in the bronchus.

Pulmonary tuberculosis is an unusual cause of cough in England. In primary tuberculosis without complicating bronchial obstruction, a cough is not to be expected. The diagnosis would be made on the history of exposure to an adult with tuberculosis (even if the tuberculosis were said to be healed), a positive tuberculin test, and x-ray of the chest, and if necessary the culture of tubercle bacilli from stomach washings.

Cough may be due to *congenital heart disease*, especially when there is a left to right shunt, or to *deficiency of alpha$_1$ antitrypsin* (Mazodier, 1970), in which there are dyspnoea, chronic antrum and respiratory infections, emphysema and sometimes hepatosplenomegaly with jaundice.

A cough may be due to a *habit, tic* or *attention-seeking device*.

Smoking must not be forgotten as a cause of chronic cough in children, and the child's cough may be due to a smoke-polluted atmosphere at home or outside in an industrial area.

References

APLEY J., LAURANCE B. & MACFATH F. (1954) Snuffles. *Lancet,* **2,** 1048.

CONNOR J.D. (1970) Etiologic rôle of adenoviral infection in pertussis syndrome. *New Engl. J. Med.,* **283,** 390.

HARRISON H.S., FUQUA W.B. & GIFFIN R.B. (1965) Congenital laryngeal cleft. *Am. J. Dis. Child.,* **110,** 556.

MAZODIER I. (1970) Hereditary deficiency of alpha₁ antitrypsin. *Pediatrie*, **6**, 7.
PYMAN C. (1971) Inhaled foreign bodies in childhood. A review of 230 cases. *Med. J. Australia*, **1**, 62.
SCHAFFER A.J. (1965) *Diseases of the Newborn*. Chicago, Saunders.

Wheezing

Wheezing is an extremely common symptom in childhood. It is commonly confused with 'ruttling'. Ruttling, heard readily without a stethoscope, is due to air bubbling through fluid in the trachea or bronchi: on auscultation coarse râles are heard. A wheeze is due to narrowing of the airway with the production of high pitched rhonchi. A wheeze nearly always signifies asthma or asthmatic bronchitis. In the first year, however, persistent 'ruttling' is commonly an early sign of asthma. On auscultation one hears some high pitched râles together with the lower pitched ones, and gradually, as the infant gets older, there is a transition to rhonchi. In an older child a ruttle is usually a sign of bronchitis but not asthma.

Asthmatic bronchitis and asthma. In the first five or perhaps six years many children respond to a cold by wheezing. One to three days after the development of a typical cold the child becomes dyspnoeic and wheezes, and the attack is indistinguishable in appearance from asthma. It is distinguished not only by the age but by the fact that there is no wheezing in between the attacks, and that the attacks never occur without a preceding cold. Even so, I would suspect that the real diagnosis was asthma if the child as a baby had eczema or if there were a strong family history of eczema or asthma.

It may be that asthmatic bronchitis is in reality an allergic condition, the cold having lowered the threshold for the allergen to cause bronchial spasm. Whatever the explanation, the prognosis for asthma and asthmatic bronchitis is different. The child with asthmatic bronchitis ceases to respond to colds by wheezing when he reaches the age of five or six: the asthmatic child is likely to continue to have attacks for many more years.

It is well known that asthma is apt to be precipitated by infections: but an asthmatic child is likely to wheeze at times when he has not just had a cold, and he is particularly liable to wheeze on exertion or on psychological stress. (The three components of asthma are allergy, infection and psychological stress.)

Wheezing may rarely be caused by enlarged *mediastinal lymph nodes*, or by a *foreign body* in the bronchus.

It is by no means easy to distinguish an asthmatic attack from laryngotracheobronchitis or bronchiolitis.

Bronchiolitis is predominantly a disease of infancy, especially of the first six months. It is usually due to the respiratory syncytial virus. The attack begins insidiously and in a day or two the child becomes severely dyspnoeic and often cyanosed. The inspiratory phase is short and expiration is prolonged. There is no stridor, but there may be a wheeze. The temperature is usually but not always raised. Bronchiolitis in infancy may be followed by asthma in later years. Wheezing is sometimes a symptom of *congenital heart disease*.

Bronchospasm is a side effect of several *drugs* and of poisoning by the organophosphorus insecticide. Drugs which may cause it include cephalosporins, erythromycin, ethionamide, lipiodol, neomycin, penicillin, rifampicin, streptomycin, tetracycline, vaccines and vitamin K.

The absence of a wheeze would eliminate asthma (except in the dangerously ill child). The absence of previous attacks would make asthma unlikely. An elevated temperature is more in favour of bronchiolitis.

Stridor

In order to consider the diagnosis, it is necessary to distinguish chronic stridor from acute stridor.

Chronic stridor

The following are the main causes to consider:

Supraglottic causes
    Congenital laryngeal stridor
    Micrognathia
    Mongolism
    Gross enlargement of tonsils and adenoids
    Lingual or laryngeal cysts (rare)
    Supraglottic webs (rare)

Glottic causes
    Laryngeal web, polyp, papilloma
    Vocal cord paralysis
    Hydrocephalus
    Foreign body
    Dislocation of the cricothyroid or cricoarytenoid articulations

Infraglottic causes
    Congenital subglottic stenosis
    Tracheal obstruction or stenosis, haemangioma, neurofibroma
    Tracheomalacia
    Vascular ring
    Mediastinal tumour or thyroid (rare)
    Foreign body

Acute stridor

Croup
Epiglottitis
Laryngitis, laryngotracheitis
Laryngitis, epiglottitis
Trauma
Foreign body
Diphtheria
Laryngeal spasm; tetany
Retropharyngeal abscess
Possibly angioneurotic oedema

Chronic stridor

The elucidation of the cause of stridor dating from birth can be a matter of considerable difficulty. It may also be a matter of great importance to the child, for some of the conditions which cause stridor may be fatal without surgical intervention. The danger of superadded upper respiratory tract infections may be considerable, and it is said by some that these children are more than usually prone to them. Hence it is important that the correct diagnosis should be known.

The first and most important observation which must be made in order to consider the diagnosis consists of the timing of the stridor. Stridor may be inspiratory or expiratory or both. *A purely inspiratory stridor is less likely to be of serious import than one which is both inspiratory and expiratory, or expiratory alone. On the other hand a purely inspiratory stridor can be due to a serious condition demanding surgical treatment.* It follows that whatever the timing of the stridor, an accurate diagnosis should be established. Stridor which is entirely inspiratory is usually of supraglottic origin. Stridor which is entirely expiratory usually arises from the trachea (Holinger & Johnston, 1955).

The second observation which must be made is the estimation of the quality of the voice. If there is hoarseness or weakness of the voice, the glottis must be involved. Severe stridor with dyspnoea, but with a normal voice, may be subglottic or tracheal in origin. Stridor with a muffled cry is likely to arise from pharyngeal or supraglottic lesions. Inspiratory stridor with an abnormal cry may be due to weakness of the recurrent laryngeal nerve or to a laryngeal web or cyst.

A high-pitched stridor persisting through inspiration or expiration usually implies severe glottic obstruction. A low-pitched stridor usually points to a supraglottic cause.

Stridor with a deep barking or 'brassy' cough usually points to tracheal obstruction.

Supraglottic causes

Supraglottic causes of stridor consist mainly of *congenital laryn-*

geal stridor (laryngomalacia) which is by far the commonest cause of stridor in infants. Other causes include *laryngeal* or *lingual cysts, supraglottic webs* and *micrognathia*.

Congenital laryngeal stridor. Congenital laryngeal stridor, the commonest cause of stridor in infants, has also been termed laryngomalacia. It dates from shortly after birth and tends to get worse until the age of three to six months. There is usually no change between the age of six and 12 months, and thereafter it usually decreases, disappearing by 18 to 24 months. It is due to abnormal collapse of the supraglottic tissues in inspiration. The epiglottis may be elongated or abnormally curved, or the arytenoepiglottic folds may be redundant. The stridor is mainly inspiratory, but is sometimes partly expiratory (Phelan *et al.* 1971). Phonation is normal. The voice and cry are unaffected. It is commonly intermittent, disappearing during rest and sleep, but much increased by crying. It is reduced in the prone position and increased when the child lies supine. The stridor is of all degrees of severity, from the most trivial to the severe. In any but the trivial degrees, there is indrawing of the lower part of the chest on inspiration.

For reasons which are not altogether clear, infants with congenital laryngeal stridor are more liable to have feeding difficulties, such as regurgitation and choking on feeding, than are normal children. I have seen most alarming cyanotic attacks in children with this condition. There is evidence that children with congenital laryngeal stridor are somewhat more likely to be mentally subnormal than others.

Apley (1953) found that seven of his 80 cases had congenital heart disease; this was regarded more as an associated finding than a cause of the stridor. He also found that there was an association between the stridor and the presence of snuffles.

Crooks (1954) regarded 90 per cent of the cases of purely inspiratory stridor as being due to laryngomalacia—an exaggeration of the infantile larynx, but ten per cent were due to other causes. He therefore advocated investigation in all cases.

Other causes of inspiratory stridor include *micrognathia, sublingual cyst* and *cysts* of the *aryepiglottic* fold. Two of Crooks' cases had a subglottic haemangioma, one had a cleft larynx, and one had a foreign body.

The micrognathic infant is liable to have inspiratory stridor, probably because the hypoplasia of the mandible permits the base of the tongue to displace the epiglottis. *Macroglossia*, seen in cretinism and other conditions, may have the same effect.

Stridor is fairly common in *mongols*. The reason is not altogether clear. In some cases seen by me lateral x-rays of the airway have demonstrated an unexplained thickening of the tissues between the vertebral column and the airway. When a child is older, stridor, worse when he is lying on his back, may be due to gross enlargement of the tonsils and adenoids. The obstruction may be so severe that it leads to cor pulmonale.

Inspiratory stridor may be due to a *thyroglossal cyst* at the base of the tongue, a *lingual thyroid* or a *dermoid cyst*. The epiglottis is pressed backwards and downwards, with the result that there is inspiratory stridor, a muffled cry and usually feeding difficulties. The condition can be demonstrated in a lateral x-ray of the airway.

A *supraglottic web* causes a marked inspiratory stridor, a subdued cry, hoarseness and chest retraction. *Laryngeal cysts* have the same effect.

Glottic lesions

Glottic lesions include in particular *laryngeal webs*, *polypi* and *papillomata*. A laryngeal web is a serious condition and the treatment is difficult. The stridor is usually but not always inspiratory only, and occurs in all positions whether the child is awake or asleep. The voice is usually abnormal and the cry weak. The diagnosis is made by laryngoscopy.

Paralysis of both vocal cords is more often seen in children with hydrocephalus, as a result of stretching of the vagi in the Arnold Chiari malformation; though hydrocephalic infants are liable to have stridor due to other but indeterminable causes. When there is bilateral cord paralysis, there is marked inspiratory stridor, chest retraction, a hoarse voice, weak cry and choking in feeds.

Stridor may be due to *birth injury*, involving damage to the recurrent laryngeal nerve, or dislocation of the cricothyroid or cricoarytenoid articulations. In either case there is hoarseness. In either case the diagnosis would be made by laryngoscopy.

Subglottic causes

Subglottic causes of stridor include in particular the *haemangioma* and *congenital subglottic stenosis*. The haemangioma causes serious obstruction, inspiratory or expiratory stridor or both, sometimes with a croupy or brassy cough. In only three of six cases described by Williams and his colleagues was there a subcutaneous naevus to provide a clue to the diagnosis. The treatment should be conservative. I have seen a case due to a *subglottic neurofibroma*. The stridor is usually inspiratory, and the cry is usually weak, but not hoarse. The diagnosis should be made by laryngoscopy and lateral x-ray.

Tracheal causes of stridor include *tracheal stenosis, tracheal cysts* and *tracheomalacia*—a condition in which there is an absence of or a defect in the cartilagenous rings. The stridor is commonly expiratory only.

An important cause of stridor is the *vascular ring*, in which there is a double aorta or an abnormally placed subclavian artery. The presenting symptom is either regurgitation of food with cyanotic attacks or stridor. The stridor is commonly both inspiratory and expiratory, but may be either inspiratory only or expiratory only. It usually occurs in sleep, as well as at rest. There is often opisthotonos, and flexion of the neck increases the dyspnoea. The cough in infants with a vascular ring is sometimes brassy or bitonal. There is unlikely to be a cardiac murmur on auscultation, or other abnormal physical signs on examination of the heart and chest. The diagnosis is made in the first place by exclusion of other causes by laryngoscopy and lateral x-ray of the airway, but it is established by x-ray of the chest with a barium swallow, followed by angiography. Some regard bronchoscopy as dangerous to these infants.

A *mediastinal tumour*, such as a thyroid, is a rare cause of stridor, but an enlarged thymus is not a cause.

In summary, there are numerous causes of chronic laryngeal stridor, most of which are amenable to surgery. Investigations needed to make the diagnosis include direct laryngoscopy, lateral x-ray of the neck to show the airway, laryngeal cinematography, an x-ray of the chest, a barium swallow and angiography.

Acute stridor

Stridor of acute origin, commonly termed *croup*, is usually due to laryngeal involvement in an acute upper respiratory tract infection, such as that due to the respiratory syncytial virus, or to laryngotracheobronchitis, which is often associated with a haemophilus influenzal infection. There are other causes such as epiglottitis, laryngeal oedema resulting from traumatic instrumentation, or a foreign body. Diphtheria is now hardly seen in the United Kingdom.

Laryngotracheobronchitis may be associated with a stridor which is inspiratory at first, and then both inspiratory and expiratory. There is indrawing of the lower part of the chest in severe cases. The air entry may be so poor that the stridor is not loud. It is by no means easy to distinguish it from asthma or acute bronchiolitis. If there is hoarseness the diagnosis of laryngotracheobronchitis is easy, but usually this is absent. One has to listen carefully in order to decide whether there is laryngitis or not. When one needs to know the diagnosis in order to decide the best line of treatment in a severely dyspnoeic child, laryngoscopy may be performed. The stridor of laryngitis could be confused with the noisy ruttle of an infant with *bronchitis* and tracheal exudate.

Acute epiglottitis may be due to haemophilus influenzae or other organisms. It occurs predominantly in the two to seven year old age group. Mild respiratory symptoms change to a severe illness, and the child rapidly becomes ill, with increasing dyspnoea from obstruction of the airway. There is a low-pitched stertor, with a louder and lower-pitched coarse expiratory rattle, resembling a snore. There may be large cervical lymph nodes, dysphagia, drooling and an intensely sore throat. The inspiratory stridor decreases as respiratory efforts increase. The voice is muffled rather than hoarse, and is therefore unlike the voice of the child with virus laryngitis. On laryngoscopy, a swollen inflamed epiglottis will be seen, but the procedure is dangerous and should only be performed by the expert with equipment for tracheostomy at hand, for it may precipitate acute obstruction. Treatment is urgent.

A mild *laryngitis* following a cold does not usually occasion anxiety; but if it occurs in a child already suffering from congenital laryngeal stridor, there are serious grounds for anxiety, because the child may rapidly develop severe dyspnoea.

Laryngeal oedema may follow *trauma* resulting from instrumentation. There is likely to be hoarseness and a croupy cough.

Laryngeal spasm may occur in *tetany*, due to hypocalcaemia resulting from rickets, coeliac disease, hypoparathyroidism or renal failure. There is a high-pitched inspiratory stridor, lasting usually for a few minutes or for a single inspiration.

A *retropharyngeal abscess* or *retropharyngeal lymphadenitis* commonly follow an upper respiratory tract infection. There is dysphagia, head retraction, mouth-breathing and fever. The abscess may be seen in the back of the throat or even felt by the finger. A lateral x-ray of the neck will show the soft tissue swelling pushing the airway forward.

References

ADDY M.G., ELLIS P.D.M., TURK D.C. (1972) Haemophilus Epiglottitis. *Brit. Med. J.*, **1**, 140.

APLEY J. (1953) The infant with stridor. *Arch. Dis. Childh.*, **28**, 423.

BENIANS R.C., BENSON P.F., SHERWOOD T. & SPECTOR R.G. (1964) Intellectual impairment in congenital laryngeal stridor. *Guy's Hosp. Rep.*, **113**, 360.

CROOKS J. (1954) Non-inflammatory laryngeal stridor in infants. *Arch. Dis. Childh.*, **29**, 11.

HOLINGER P.H. & JOHNSTON K.C. (1955) The infant with respiratory stridor. *Pediat. Clinics. N. Am.*, May, p. 403.

MACARTNEY F.J., PANDAY J. & SCOTT O. (1960) Cor pulmonale as a result of nasopharyngeal obstruction due to hypertrophied tonsils and adenoids. *Arch. Dis. Childh.*, **44**, 585.

PHELAN P.D., GILLAM G.L., STOCKS J.G., WILLIAMS H.E. (1971) The Clinical and Physiological manifestation of the Infantile Larynx. *Australian Paediat. J.*, **7**, 135.

PRACY R. (1965) Stridor in children. *Proc. Roy. Soc. Med.*, **58**, 267.

SCHAFFER A.J. (1960) *Diseases of the Newborn*. Philadelphia, Saunders.

WILLIAMS H.E., PHELAN P.D., STOCKS J.G., WOOD H. (1969) Haemangiomas of larynx in Infants. *Australian Paediat. J.*, **5**, 149.

Chest pain

The most frequent cause of chest pain is stitch; this is a cramp-like pain on one side of the lower part of the chest or upper part of the abdomen, occurring on exertion after a meal. It is probably due to strain on the peritoneal ligaments attached to the diaphragm.

Pleural friction or pleural pain causes a knife-like stabbing pain, worse on respiration or coughing. The usual causes are pneumonia or epidemic pleurodynia (Bornholm disease).

An unrecognised *injury*, such as a fractured rib, should be considered as a possible cause.

Pericarditis may result from rheumatic fever, tuberculosis, pyogenic organisms or a virus infection (e.g. coxsackie virus).

True *angina* is a rare symptom, occurring in association with rheumatic disease of the aortic valves.

Acute shoulder-tip pain should suggest pleural friction or referred pain from a *ruptured spleen.*

Reference

ABRAHAMS A. (1959) Stitch. *Practitioner*, **182,** 771.

Haemoptysis

Haemoptysis is an unusual symptom in childhood. It is most unlikely to be due to tuberculosis. It hardly ever occurs in primary tuberculosis, but could occur in the adult type of tuberculosis in the older child. It is unusual in lobar pneumonia.

It is frequently not easy to decide whether blood has been brought up from the chest or from the stomach (e.g. after a nose bleed).

Causes of haemoptysis include:

Blood diseases
Whooping cough

Trauma (e.g. a broken rib)
Foreign body in the lung
Bronchiectasis
Heart failure
Uraemia
Bronchial polyp
Pulmonary abscess
Malignant disease
Pulmonary haemosiderosis (rare)

The importance of blood diseases when there is unexplained haemoptysis must be emphasised. The possibility of a foreign body must never be forgotten in many obscure pulmonary conditions in children.

Red colouration of the sputum results from the taking of rifampicin.

Dyspnoea

Dyspnoea of acute onset, without significant previous symptoms, is likely to be due to pneumonia, asthma, asthmatic bronchitis, foreign body in the airpassage, pneumothorax, mediastinal or obstructive emphysema, a massive collapse of the lung, large air containing cyst, pleural effusion, pericarditis or heart failure (due to paroxysmal tachycardia or congenital heart disease). Paroxysmal tachycardia is readily missed in an infant. It usually masquerades as bronchopneumonia, on account of the rapid breathing and cough due to heart failure.

Chronic dyspnoea may be due to the following conditions:

Chest conditions
  Asthma
  Unrecognised pleural effusion
  Obstructive emphysema
  Large air-containing cyst
  Pneumothorax

Massive collapse of lung
Pulmonary agenesis
Pulmonary fibrosis, cor pulmonale, aspergillosis, Farmer's lung
Diaphragmatic hernia
Mediastinal mass
Alpha$_1$ antitrypsin deficiency
Heart conditions
  Congenital heart disease
  Rheumatic heart disease
  Adherent pericardium
Skeletal conditions
  Severe chest deformity

Anaemia

Obesity

Abdominal conditions—ascites

Renal failure

Drugs

It is one of the characteristic features of *asthma* that exertion causes wheezing and therefore dyspnoea. In severe cases the emphysema causes dyspnoea on exertion.

One has seen children referred for breathlessness with an unrecognised *pleural effusion* or large *diaphragmatic hernia*.

Obstructive emphysema, due to a tuberculous lymph node, a foreign body or other lesion, may cause symptoms and signs similar to those of a large air-containing cyst or pneumothorax.

Serious progressive dyspnoea results from *pulmonary fibrosis* and especially from *fibrocystic disease of the pancreas*. A common end result of fibrocytic disease of the pancreas or extensive bronchiectasis is cor pulmonale with severe dyspnoea. Another cause of severe extensive fibrosis is the *Hamman-Rich syndrome*. The Hamman-Rich syndrome consists of diffuse interstitial fibrosis of the lungs, and leads to progressive dyspnoea and death. The diagnosis is made by x-ray. *Pulmonary aspergillosis* should be considered when there is asthma and eosinophilia: it is diagnosed by a skin test and serological methods. *Farmer's lung* is associated with the inhalation of the dust of mouldy vegetable material: it is associated with malaise, fever, febrile aches and pains and dyspnoea. It is diagnosed by the presence of precipitins in the serum. Alpha₁ antitrypsin deficiency may present as unexplained dyspnoea (p. 143).

Congenital heart disease, and especially pulmonary stenosis (with or without Fallot's tetralogy), is perhaps the commonest cause of chronic breathlessness in the first three or four years. After the age of four or five, severe rheumatic carditis is a possible but unusual cause of chronic breathlessness. An *adherent pericardium* is another possible cause.

Severe chest deformity, such as that associated with kyphosis or severe degrees of funnel chest, may cause breathlessness. Severe anaemia or ascites are other causes. Renal failure with uraemia or hypertension are other possibilities.

Dyspnoea may be a side effect of rifampicin.

References

BRADLEY C.A. (1956) Diffuse interstitial fibrosis of the lungs in children. *J. Pediat.*, **48,** 442.

PEPYS J. (1965) Hypersensitivity reactions in relation to pulmonary fibrosis. *La Medicina del Lavoro*, **56,** 451 (in English).

Overventilation

Overventilation in older children, over the age of six or seven, may be *hysterical* and progress to tetany. It may be due to *diabetic acidosis, uraemia, metabolic acidosis in gastroenteritis*, or *drugs*, notably acetazolamide, aminophylline, salicylates or sulthiame. Salicylate poisoning is an important cause of overventilation, and must be considered however firmly the parents deny that the child has had access to the drug. They may deny the possibility because they do not wish to admit that they have been careless in the storage of drugs, or because they genuinely do not know that the child obtained the drug, or because they deliberately left the drug in an accessible place (child abuse). The diagnosis is confirmed by the phenistix test and subsequently by estimation of the serum salicylate level. The characteristic feature is deep heavy breathing. The diagnosis is confirmed by the phenistix test and by a serum salicylate estimation.

Sulthiame (Ospolot), used for the treatment of epilepsy, *aminophylline* used for the treatment of asthma, and *acetazolamide*, may cause overventilation.

Diabetic acidosis and *uraemia* are other important causes of overventilation. The former would be readily diagnosed by the smell of acetone in the breath and the finding of glycosuria.

Reference

PICKERING D. (1964) Salicylate poisoning. The diagnosis when its possibility is denied by the parents. *Acta Paediat. Uppsala,* **53,** 501.

Blurring of vision and diplopia

When a child who has previously had normal vision complains of continuous blurring of vision, careful examination and investigation are essential. The causes include the following:

Error of refraction
Papilloedema or field of vision defect, due to a cerebral tumour or
        abscess, or a demyelinating disease of the nervous system
Iridocyclitis or other inflammatory condition of the eye
Cataract
Mucus in association with conjunctivitis or with a Meibomian cyst
        on the eyelid
The effect of drugs
Psychological causes, including hysteria
    Other causes of diplopia include *iridocyclitis* or *cataract*. Cataracts

may be of prenatal origin (maternal rubella or genetic), or acquired. They are common in mongols and may result from corticosteroid therapy.

Iridocyclitis may commence with an *eye injury*, a *foreign body* or *infection*. It occurs in about ten per cent of children with *rheumatoid arthritis*. It is a common sequel of *congenital syphilis*.

When one has eliminated the obvious causes of blurring of vision, the refraction of the eye should be tested by an ophthalmologist.

A *Meibomian* cyst on the eyelid may lead to the formation of mucus which alters the refraction of the eye and leads to blurring with unilateral diplopia.

A variety of *drugs* may cause blurring of vision. They include amitriptyline, antihistamines, barbiturates, capreomycin, carbamazepine, chloramphenicol, cloroquine, ethambutol, gentamycin, imipramine, indomethacin, isoniazid, kanamycin, meprobamate, nalidixic acid, PAS, phenothiazines, piperazine, primidone, sulphonamides, sulthiame, tetracycline and troxidone. Glue sniffing may cause blurring of vision. The antihistamines, phenytoin, primidone and nalidixic acid may cause diplopia.

Corticosteroids, chlorambucil and indomethacin may lead to cataract formation, and chloroquine may cause corneal opacities and retinal damage.

Chloramphenicol may cause optic neuritis.

Ethambutol and capreomycin may cause loss of colour vision, and digoxin may cause xanthopsia.

Blurring of vision may be entirely *psychological*. It may be due to neurosis, malingering or hysteria. These diagnoses are dangerous ones, and it is essential that one should be sure that there is no organic disease and that there is positive evidence of psychological disturbance.

Blindness or severe defect of vision

It is not easy to assess the vision of an infant in the early weeks. In mentally defective infants it is often impossible for several weeks or months to assess the visual acuity. It is easy to make the mistake of considering that the child is blind, because he does not seem to take any interest in objects, when in fact his lack of interest is due to mental deficiency. As he matures it becomes clear that he can see. The optic disc of normal babies is pale, and it is easy to make the mistaken diagnosis of optic atrophy when in fact the discs are normal.

The most important indication of a visual defect in a baby is a roving nystagmus. By simple developmental testing after the mental age of about four months one can obtain some idea of whether the child can see.

The following conditions increase the risk that a child will have a visual defect:

Family history
Prematurity (retrolental fibroplasia, cataract, myopia, squint)
Rubella in early pregnancy
Mental deficiency
Toxaemia in pregnancy
Hydrocephalus, craniostenosis
Ophthalmia neonatorum
Cerebral palsy
Squint
Suppression of squinting eye
Drugs
Trauma—airgun, catapult, bows and arrows, fireworks
  Indelible pencil

Rare
  Metabolic diseases—cystinosis, Lowe's syndrome, Marfan's disease
  Rheumatoid arthritis
  Cytomegalovirus infection and toxoplasmosis

Prematurity predisposes to visual defects for various reasons. One is the risk of retrolental fibroplasia if an excess of oxygen is used. Other conditions with which prematurity is associated include myopia, strabismus and cataract.

Severe *toxaemia* or *hypertension* in pregnancy predisposes to myopia.

Rubella in the first three months of pregnancy may lead to cataract, deafness, congenital heart disease, mental deficiency, thrombocytopenic purpura, hepatitis or other defects in the foetus.

There is a fairly strong association between *mental deficiency* and the various eye defects. This is partly due to the fact that optic atrophy is commonly associated with mental subnormality.

If a *squint* is not corrected by the age of about nine to 12 months, the child will suppress the squinting eye and become blind in it.

Certain rare *metabolic diseases* may be associated with visual defects: they include cystinosis (in which one sign is rickets), Lowe's syndrome (in which the eye and kidney are affected), and Marfan's disease (in which there is arachnodactyly and dislocation of the lens).

Rheumatoid arthritis is followed or accompanied in some ten per cent of cases by iridocyclitis.

Various *drugs*, such as chloramphenicol or isoniazid, may cause optic astrophy.

Optic neuritis may be due to neuromyelitis optica—in which the child develops transverse myelitis and optic neuritis, with loss of tendon reflexes.

A child may lose his vision for a short period only at the beginning of an attack of *migraine*.

Certain rare *vascular disorders* are associated with loss of vision: they include arteriovenous malformation and central retinal artery occlusion.

Reference

ILLINGWORTH R.S. (1972) *Development of the Infant and Young Child, Normal and Abnormal*. Edinburgh, Churchill Livingstone.

Nystagmus

By far the commonest cause of nystagmus in an infant is a defect of vision such as optic atrophy. This should be considered to be the diagnosis until proved otherwise. The nystagmus in such children is often but not always of the roving type, unlike the finer nystagmus due to other conditions.

The following are the main causes of nystagmus:

Defect of vision and astigmatism
Congenital nystagmus
Anti-epileptic and other drugs
Albinism
Spasmus nutans
Cerebellar ataxia
Friedreich's ataxia
Cerebellar tumour or abscess

Various *drugs* can cause nystagmus. They include in particular anticonvulsants, colistin, diphenoxylate and salicylates.

Nystagmus is almost invariable in *albinism*, and it is usual in *spasmus nutans* (p. 183), in which there are jerky head movements, ceasing when the child concentrates on an object.

Nystagmus may be caused by various diseases of the cerebellum or cerebellar tracts—such as Friedreich's ataxia, congenital ataxia, tumour or abscess. *Friedreich's ataxia* is a progressive hereditary disease, whose features include ataxia, absence of the knee jerks, plantar extensor responses and pes cavus with Rombergism.

Retinal haemorrhages

For retinal haemorrhages in the newborn see p. 53.

Large retinal haemorrhages are usually found in the presence of a *subdural haematoma.*

They may result from *head injury, severe whooping cough,* or from *blood diseases.*

Lachrymation

The eye-watering of the young infant (epiphora) is not strictly lachrymation; it is due to delay in the opening of the nasolachrymal duct.

Lachrymation may result from any painful injury or disease of the eye, including a foreign body. Phlyctenular conjunctivitis due to tuberculosis may be a cause. It may be due to any disease of the lachrymal gland and occasionally to eyestrain. It has been described in thyrotoxicosis.

Lachrymation may be a side effect of nitrazepam or iodides.

Strabismus

It is essential that a squint should be diagnosed shortly after the age of six months, because if left untreated the child will develop amblyopia as a result of suppressing the squinting eye. It is normal for some degree of strabismus to occur before the age of six months but a fixed squint at any age is always abnormal, so that the child should be referred to an ophthalmologist as soon as possible. A fixed squint is commonly found in cerebral palsy, microcephaly and hydrocephalus. The rapid development of a squint may suggest the possibility of a cerebral tumour. An important and treatable condition which causes a fixed squint in the first few weeks is the retinoblastoma.

Squints are due to imbalance of muscle, as a result of weakness or maldevelopment of the muscle or faulty innervation; to differences in the refraction of the two eyes; to hypermetropia or to visual defect in one eye—such as that due to a corneal opacity. There is a somewhat increased incidence of squints in premature born or clumsy children. There is often a family history of the same complaint. A squint is an unusual side effect of *nalidixic acid*.

A false appearance of a convergent squint is caused by *epicanthic folds*.

When the squint is of the paralytic type (non-comitant), due to paralysis of muscle, the eyes are straight except when moved in the direction of the paralysed muscle, when diplopia occurs.

When the squint is concomitant (non-paralytic), as it usually is, all muscles move the eye normally, but they do not work in conjunction with each other. The two eyes are in the same relative position to each other whatever the direction of the gaze. There is no diplopia.

In young infants one can determine whether there is a squint by noting the position of the light reflex on each cornea when a torch is held in front of the child. The reflex in each eye should be in the centre of the pupil or at a corresponding point on the two corneas.

In testing an older child, one covers one eye while with the other he looks at a light. When the card is slowly moved away, the eyes should not move if the eyes are straight. If there is esotropia, the eyes will both move outwards to fix on the light; if there is exotropia (divergent), each eye will move inward to fix on the light. The examiner watches the eye which is being uncovered.

Ptosis

The commonest cause of ptosis in a child is a hereditary one.

The principal causes of ptosis are as follows:

Congenital or hereditary

Rare
  Congenital facial diplegia (Möbius syndrome)
  Oculomotor nerve paralysis
  Myasthenia gravis (p. 38).

Horner's syndrome
Dystropic ophthalmoplegia
Jaw winking (Marcus Gunn phenomenon)
Tumours
Myotubular myopathy
Drugs

In *congenital ptosis* there is defective development or absence of the levator palpebrae superioris or defect of the superior rectus. The condition may be hereditary.

Ptosis may be a feature of both the Möbius syndrome (congenital facial diplegia, p. 207) and myotonia dystrophica (p. 207). In both there is a characteristic immobile face with open mouth.

Oculomotor nerve paralysis occurs without known cause, possibly as a result of agenesis of the nerve or nucleus.

Horner's syndrome consists of a disturbance of the cervical sympathetic chain, leading to unilateral meiosis, apparent enophthalmos, ptosis and absence of facial sweating.

Dystrophic ophthalmoplegia may start at any time from infancy to adult life, usually with ptosis as the first symptom. It is slowly progressive, and is confined to the levators of the eyelid and the external ocular muscles. Later there is weakness of the lateral and vertical movements of the eyes.

In the *Marcus Gunn phenomenon* there is ptosis until the mouth is opened, when the eyelid is simultaneously raised.

An important cause of ptosis in early childhood is a ***neuroblastoma*** with deposits in the orbit.

A rare form of *myopathy* ('myotubular') is associated with ptosis.

The drug *vincristine* may cause ptosis.

Proptosis

Proptosis is an uncommon symptom of childhood. The usual causes are as follows:

Craniostenosis
Craniofacial dysostosis

Neuroblastoma or other tumour of the eye or orbit
Orbital haemorrhage, leukaemia, pertussis
Orbital cellulitis
Cavernous sinus thrombosis
Thyrotoxicosis
Aneurism

Craniofacial dysostosis (Crouzon's disease) is a rare condition in which there is a small maxilla, a beak-shaped nose, acrocephaly, protruding lower lip and exophthalmos.

Tumours of the eye or orbit which cause ptosis include the dermoid, orbital encephalocele, teratoma, glioma, haemangioma, neuroblastoma, neurofibroma, osteoma, rhabdomyosarcoma, mucocele of the paranasal sinus, histiocytosis x.

Orbital cellulitis can readily be confused with cavernous sinus thrombosis. The latter is usually secondary to infection around the orbit or face. There are rigors and fever, and the child is ill. The signs are usually more localised in the case of orbital cellulitis.

Orbital haemorrhage may occur in blood diseases and in severe pertussis.

A rare cause of proptosis is an aneurism. Auscultation of the eye may reveal a continuous systolic murmur.

Photophobia

By far the commonest cause of photophobia used to be *Pink Disease*, due to mercury intoxication. This is not seen now.

Photophobia may be a manifestation of *meningitis, measles, albinism* and *Vitamin A deficiency*.

It may be a side effect of *troxidone* or P.A.S.

It is a troublesome symptom in *phlyctenular conjunctivitis*, which is usually due to tuberculosis; there are white or grey papules 1–2 mm in diameter on the cornea or bulbar conjunctiva, with injection of the surrounding sclera. There may be profuse lachrymation.

Myopia

The following are the known causes of myopia:

Congenital and familial. Myopia is commonly a familial feature. There may be other congenital conditions, such as colobomata or albinism

Maternal toxaemia or hypertension. A history of these conditions is frequent when myopia is severe

Malnutrition in utero. Prematurity and particularly dysmaturity are common precursors. Retrolental *fibroplasia* may be associated with myopia

Social. Myopia is more common in the poor than in the well to do

Degenerative conditions, usually commencing after the age of four. They may lead to retinal degeneration or detachment of the retina

The effect of drugs (rare). These include tetracycline, sulphonamides and acetazolamide

Reference

GARDINER P. & JAMES G. (1960) Myopia. *Br. J. Ophthal.,* 44, 172.

Ear pain

The usual causes of ear pain are otitis media or a boil in the external auditory meatus. Other causes include an erupting or carious molar tooth, herpes of the external auditory meatus, otitis externa or pain referred from the throat or larynx. A foreign body in the ear might cause pain.

Defective hearing

A child may appear to be deaf because he does not listen—perhaps because he is engrossed in an interesting occupation, or because of indiscipline or bad manners. A mentally defective child is apt to be slow to respond to sound and to be wrongly suspected of deafness.

A child with infantile autism may appear to be deaf because of lack of social responsiveness.

If a parent suspects deafness it is quite likely that her fears are well founded, and a full testing should always be carried out by an expert.

Conditions which increase the risk that a child will have a defect of hearing include the following:

Deafness suspected by parents
Plug of wax in the ear
Family history
Maternal rubella in first three months
Hyperbilirubinaemia in the newborn
Prematurity, especially extreme
Severe anoxia at birth
Recurrent otitis. Adenoids
Cleft palate
Delayed or defective speech
Cerebral palsy, especially athetosis
Mental subnormality
Drugs
Meningitis
Cretinism

Rare
    Congenital nephritis
    Waardenburg's syndrome (white forelock, etc.)
    Treacher-Collins syndrome
    Klippel-Feil syndrome

Retinitis pigmentosa

Acoustic neuroma

Osteogenesis imperfecta

Before other factors are considered one should examine the ears with an auriscope in order to eliminate blockage of the meatus by wax.

There may be a family history of *congenital deafness*. This has to be distinguished from deafness acquired as a result of otitis media and other causes.

About 30 per cent of children born by mothers who had *rubella* in the first three months of pregnancy will have some defect of hearing. It should be noted that this may be only partial or it may be confined to one ear.

Hyperbilirubinaemia in the newborn period, whether due to prematurity, haemolytic disease or other causes, predisposes to deafness. In the fully-developed case there are other signs of kernicterus such as athetosis. A history of severe jaundice in the newborn period should alert one to the possibility of deafness in later months and years.

There is some association between deafness and premature delivery or severe anoxia at birth.

Cerebral palsy and *mental abnormality* are strongly associated with deafness. Some 20 to 25 per cent of all children with cerebral palsy have some degree of deafness. Children with athetosis are more likely to have a hearing defect than those with the spastic form of cerebral palsy.

A variety of *drugs* cause deafness. Some of these may affect the child when given to the pregnant woman. The main ones are capreomycin, colistin, dihydrostreptomycin, framycetin, frusemide, gentamicin, kanamycin, neomycin, nortriptyline, paromomycin, quinine, salicylates, streptomycin, vancomycin, vincristine and viomycin.

Meningitis and *recurrent otitis* are important causes of deafness. The danger that recurrent attacks of otitis may cause deafness, particularly if perforation of the drum is allowed to occur, is an important reason for the prompt treatment of otitis media. The development of deafness in association with a mass of adenoids is a strong indication for adenoidectomy.

Many children with a *cleft palate* develop deafness in later years, for reasons not altogether understood.

A variety of congenital syndromes are associated with deafness. They include *hereditary nephritis, cretinism, Waardenburg's syndrome,* the *Treacher-Collins* and the *Klippel-Feil syndrome* and *retinitis pigmentosa.* Waardenburg's syndrome consists of a white forelock, an unequal colour of the iris of the two eyes (heterochromia), and congenital deafness. The Treacher-Collins syndrome consists of a gross deformity of the ears, a small lower jaw and cleft palate, with other deformities of the face. The Klippel-Feil syndrome consists of a congenital abnormality and fusion of the cervical vertebrae. Retinitis pigmentosa can easily be missed if not looked for; it consists of multiple small patches of pigmentation in the retina.

Conclusion

There are many possible causes of deafness and many factors which increase the likelihood of deafness. These 'risk' factors should alert one to the possibility of deafness. It must be remembered that the child born with defective hearing cannot know that he does not hear well. It is our responsibility to make the diagnosis. Every child with delayed or defective speech much have his hearing tested by an expert.

The method of diagnosis has been described in detail in my book (Illingworth, 1972). Suitable test sounds are the crinkling of paper, a small hand bell, the sound PS or PHTH (for high tones) and oo (for low tones), on a level with the ear and 12 to 18 inches away, out of sight of the baby. In the first three months the baby may respond by a startle reflex, by blinking the eyes, by crying, or by quieting if he is already crying. Between three and four months he begins to respond by turning his head to sound.

References

ARTHUR L.J.H. (1965) Some hereditary syndromes that include deafness. *Develop. Med. Child Neurol.*, **7**, 395.

ILLINGWORTH R.S. (1972) *Development of the Infant and Young Child. Normal and Abnormal.* Edinburgh, Churchill Livingstone.

Tinnitus

The complaint of buzzing in the ears (tinnitus) may be purely psychological.

Tinnitus is caused by certain drugs, especially salicylates and quinine.

The symptom may originate from an acoustic nerve tumour.

A rare cause is an intracranial arteriovenous communication. It is worth while looking for distended veins on the face and scalp, and auscultating the skull for a continuous bruit.

Vertigo

Vertigo is such a subjective symptom that it is not easy to assess it in children. Vertigo commonly precedes a faint or fit, or occurs with a change of posture, especially when the child has been or is unwell or is anaemic.

Other causes include:

Epidemic vertigo
Benign paroxysmal vertigo
Drugs
Cerebellar lesions
Acoustic neuroma
Labyrinthitis after mumps
Posterior fossa tumour
Chronic otitis media
Ramsay Hunt syndrome (facial palsy with herpes of the external auditory canal)
Hypoglycaemia
Occlusive disease of the vertebrobasilar vessels

Epidemic vertigo is probably a virus infection. The onset is usually sudden, with nausea or vomiting. It may be associated with nystagmus and diplopia. It usually lasts for a few days only and is apparently infectious.

Benign paroxysmal vertigo is a mysterious but distressing condition, occurring mainly in early childhood, in which there is a sudden attack of severe vertigo lasting for seconds or minutes. The child is often terrified, becomes pale, sweats and may vomit. It can readily be mistaken for an epileptic fit. The attacks may recur after an interval of days or months. They cease after a period varying from four months to four years. It is possible that they are a form of Menière's disease and tests may reveal abnormal vestibular function. For acute ataxia see p. 175.

Rare cases of vertigo include *cerebellar tumour and abscess*, and the *acoustic neuroma, labyrinthitis* complicating mumps, a *posterior fossa tumour, chronic otitis media* and the *Ramsay-Hunt syndrome* (facial palsy with herpes of the external auditory canal), hypoglycaemia and occlusive disease of the vertebrobasilar vessels. In the latter condition there are attacks of vertigo, followed later by the development of ataxia. Diagnosis is by vertebral angiography.

Vertigo may be due to certain *drugs*, especially acetazolamide, amitriptyline, antihistamines, carbamazepine, colistin, diazepam, gentamicin, griseofulvin, imipramine, indomethacin, isoniazid, kanamycin, meprobamate, nalidixic acid, paromomycin, pethidine, phenytoin, phenothiazines, phensuccimide, piperazine, polymyxin, primidone, salicylates, sulphonamides, thiazides, thiobendazole and trimethoprim.

References

Basser L.S. (1964) Benign paroxysmal vertigo of childhood (a variety of vestibular neuronitis). *Brain*, 87, 141.

Cawthorne T. (1952) Vertigo. *Brit. med. J.*, 2, 931.

Harvey C.C. (1967) Paroxysmal vertigo in children. *Arch. Dis. Childh.*, 42, 564.

Koenigsberger M.R., Chutorian A.M., Gold A. & Schvey M.S. (1970). Paroxysmal vertigo of childhood. *Neurology* 22, 1108.

Leishman A.W.D. (1955) Epidemic vertigo with oculomotor complications. *Lancet*, 1, 228.

The clumsy child

The following conditions have to be considered:

Delayed motor maturation. Familial
Normal variation
Emotional factors
Mental subnormality
Minimal cerebral dysfunction
    Minimal cerebral palsy of the spastic, ataxic or athetoid type
    Tremor
    Difficulty in spatial appreciation
Chorea
The effect of drugs
Mirror movements
Klippel-Feil syndrome
Muscular dystrophy
Degenerative diseases of the nervous system
Cerebral tumours
Riley's syndrome

    The child who was late in learning to walk will be late in learning to walk steadily, and will fall much more than others of the same age who learnt to walk sooner.

    Mothers commonly complain that one of their children falls a great deal, always has bruises on his legs, or seems awkward with his hands. The teacher is apt to complain that such a child writes badly, holds his pencil in an odd way and is poor at physical training. Such children may have difficulty in tying shoe-laces or buttoning coats. They may swing the arms in an odd way, bump into furniture, misjudge distance (as in going through a doorway) and frequently break objects. They find needle threading a hopeless task: they are awkward in dressing, drawing, writing or feeding themselves. They tend to write with the whole body, with the tongue protruding and the paper at an unusual angle, while the free hand roams. They sometimes have difficulty in distinguishing right from left. They cannot throw a ball properly. These children often concentrate badly and are overactive and impulsive. They commonly find reading difficult and may indulge in mirror writing. They may have difficulties in spatial appreciation. All the symptoms are made worse by scolding. Affected children commonly present as behaviour problems. They get into constant trouble at school, for teachers are apt to think that they are just naughty, dull, lazy or awkward. They may present as truancy. They often hate games because they are so bad at them and are therefore apt to be unpopular and to be ridiculed by their fellows. They are liable to develop various manifestations of insecurity, such as stuttering, excessive shyness, silly behaviour or bed-wetting.

On superficial examination these children look normal and intelligent. They may have an IQ well above the average, though some are merely average or below average. On careful neurological examination some abnormal signs may be found. Whereas a normal child of three can stand for a few seconds and at four quite steadily on one foot, many of the clumsy children at the age of five, six or seven or so are unsteady when standing on one foot. They cannot jump like a three-year-old or hop like a five-year-old. When building a tower of ten cubes they are apt to have some tremor of the hand and so knock the tower down accidentally before it is completed. In timed tests of fine manipulation, such as the placing of small pegs into a peg board, they are far below the average in performance. They are poor at placing shaped objects through holes or at making designs with blocks or at copying letters. In the various tests performed by the psychologist, the performance is much inferior to the verbal tests.

There are wide normal variations in children, and these variations are often familial. Sometimes they are of emotional origin and are related to insecurity, yet many 'clumsy' children, though regarded as 'normal' but 'naughty' by their teachers, are not really normal—they have evidence of organic disease.

Mentally subnormal children tend to be more clumsy with the hands and other movements than normal children.

The term *'minimal cerebral dysfunction'*, suggested in the excellent symposium edited by Bax and MacKeith is a good descriptive term, in that it does not attempt to give a precise diagnosis. It is wrong to use the term 'birth injury' for these children, because there is no evidence that their troubles are due to birth injury. The term 'brain damage' is apt to be thought synonymous with 'birth injury', though some intend the term to refer to the prenatal period as well as to the event of birth. It is known that these symptoms are relatively common in infants born prematurely, and Knobloch and Pasamanick found some relation between the symptoms and maternal toxaemia and hypertension. Prechtl in Holland found that undue irritability or drowsiness at birth was liable to be followed in later years by overactivity, clumsiness and poor concentration. It may be a sequel of neonatal hyperbilirubinaemia.

In some of these children there are minimal signs of the *spastic variety of cerebral palsy*. In some there is merely ataxia; they are examples of 'congenital ataxia'. In some there are minimal signs of the athetoid form of cerebral palsy. Some have a slight tremor which interferes with fine hand movements. In fact it is probable that the clinical picture is the end result of several pathological processes. Sometimes the problem is one of difficulty in spatial appreciation.

Awkwardness and clumsiness with poor writing and emotional disturbance are common features of early *chorea*, and should always alert one to the possibility of chorea if the child had been normal previously. *Anti-epileptic drugs*, in particular phenytoin, commonly cause ataxia when the blood level rises about 3 mg per cent.

Some children are clumsy because of *mirror movements*. When one hand tries to get a button through a button hole, the opposite free hand makes the same movements. As a result of these mirror movements the child finds it difficult to tie shoe-laces and to carry out innumerable daily tasks.

Some children with the *Klippel-Feil* syndrome have a similar difficulty. They cannot let go of something with one hand while grasping with the other. This makes it difficult to climb a ladder.

Muscular dystrophy is an important cause of awkwardness of movement and frequent falling. In the common Duchenne variety there is particular difficulty in climbing stairs. Serum enzyme tests will clinch the diagnosis if it is in doubt. There is a rare form of congenital myopathy which is manifested by persistent clumsiness.

A wide variety of degenerative diseases of the nervous system, such as *Friedreich's ataxia*, cause clumsiness. A *cerebral tumour* may present as ataxia. A rare cause of clumsiness is *Riley's syndrome* (p. 40).

Conclusion

It is well worth while referring a 'clumsy' child to an expert, because the diagnosis can be difficult and there are many possible causes to consider. The important thing is to establish the fact that there really is organic disease and therefore a good reason for his awkwardness.

For References, see p. 178.

Ataxia

Ataxia may be caused by a variety of conditions including the following:

Drugs
Friedreich's ataxia (161)
Cerebral tumour
Ataxia telangiectasia
Acute cerebellar ataxia
Heat stroke
Hypothyroidism syndrome
Abetalipoproteinaemia
Hartnup disease
Maple syrup urine disease
Pelizaeus Merzbacher disease
Disseminated sclerosis
Refsum's syndrome

A variety of *drugs* cause ataxia—in particular amitriptyline, antihistamines, chlordiazepoxide, colistin, cyclopentolate, diazepam, diphenoxylate, indomethacin, meprobamate, nitrazepam, pheneturide, phensuccimide, phenytoin, piperazine, polymyxin, primidone, streptomycin, sulthiame and vincristine. *Glue sniffing* and *alcohol* may cause severe ataxia.

Solvent sniffing amongst school children and adolescents is a serious problem in Canada and the United States. It behoves all of us to remember its possibility in Great Britain. Fumes from glues and plastic cements used in ready made building kits, aeroplane glues, lacquer enamels, nail polish remover, paint thinners, contain such substances as benzene, carbon tetrachloride, toluene, xylene, alcohol, acetone and amylacetate; and gasoline contains naphtha. All these substances are CNS depressants. They may arouse a feeling of exhilaration, but later ataxia, diplopia or confusion may arise. It is said to be common in New York slums.

Because of the possibility of a *cerebral tumour or abscess*, the fundi must always be examined for papilloedema.

Ataxia telangiectasia is a hereditary condition with telangiectasia of the skin and conjunctiva, progressive ataxia, nasal discharge, athetosis and reduced resistance to infection.

Blau and Sheehan have described a condition rather similar to that of epidemic vertigo. Children aged one to four, commonly seven to ten days after a respiratory infection, develop *acute ataxia*, reaching a maximum in 24 to 72 hours. The cerebrospinal fluid is normal, or contains a few cells. Recovery is complete in days or weeks. The condition may be due to infectious mononucleosis or to encephalitis.

Heat stroke is a possible cause of acute ataxia.

Hagberg and Westphal described an ataxic syndrome associated with *hypothyroidism*. Another rare cause is *abetalipoproteinaemia*. Progressive ataxia may be caused by a *posterior fossa tumour*.

Ataxia is a feature of abetalipoproteinaemia (p. 12). In *Hartnup disease* there are episodes of ataxia with pellagra-like skin lesions. In *maple syrup urine disease* there are episodes of ataxia and convulsions, and the urine smells of maple syrup. The *Pelizaeus Merzbacher syndrome* is a sex-linked slowly degenerative disease with nystagmus, ataxia, tremors and spasticity. *Disseminated sclerosis* may commence in childhood. *Refsum's syndrome* is characterised by ichthyosis, the development of nerve deafness at about four to eight years of age, retinitis pigmentosa, ataxia and mental deterioration.

For References, see p. 178.

Overactivity

It is difficult to define the term overactivity with any precision. Many mothers think that their children are 'overactive', and complain that they are always on the go and never sit still, when in fact they are normal. This sort of behaviour is usual in the child from five to ten or so. The healthy six-year-old is always on the go: he does not walk, he runs; when his mother holds one hand he skips and hops. What is normal at one age, however, is not normal at another. As children mature they lose much of this excessive activity. In this section I will discuss what one may term 'unusual overactivity'. This is commonly accompanied by lack of concentration, ready distractability and short attention span. The children tend to be impulsive, clumsy, excessively talkative and even destructive. Their movements are more purposeless than just increased in amount. These children wear their mothers out and exhaust their teachers.

The main causes of 'unusual overactivity' may be summarised as follows:

Heredity
Personality
Excessive restraint
Insecurity
Mental subnormality
Autism
Temporal lobe epilepsy
'Minimal cerebral dysfunction'
The effect of drugs

Unusual overactivity may be a *familial* trait. It may be partly a matter of an inherited personality characteristic. It must not be

assumed that an overactive child has suffered 'brain injury' with
out first enquiring about the behaviour of the mother or father a
that age.

Mental subnormality is a common cause of unusual overactivity
in the young child, partly because mentally subnormal children
mature more slowly than normal ones. As a result they are late in
growing out of the overactivity of the normal young child. An
autistic child may show troublesome overactivity. Overactivity may
be a complication of *temporal lobe epilepsy*.

Excessive *restraint*, possibly by causing insecurity, directly or in
directly may be a cause of unusual overactivity.

For *'minimal cerebral dysfunction'* see p. 173.

For *chorea* and other forms of involuntary movement, see the
next section.

Certain *drugs* may be responsible for overactivity. They include
chlordiazepoxide, phenobarbitone and primidone.

References

Bax M. & MacKeith R. (1963) Minimal cerebral dysfunction. *Little Club
Clin. Dev. Med. No. 10.*

Blau M.E. & Sheehan J.C. (1968) Acute cerebellar syndrome of childhood
Neurology, **8**, 538.

Glaser H.H. & Masengale O.N. (1962) Glue sniffing in children. *J. Am
med. Ass.*, **181**, 300.

Hagberg B. & Westphal O. (1970) Ataxic syndrome in congenital hypothyroidism. *Acta. Paediat. Scandinav.*, **59**, 323.

Hatton D.E. (1966) The child with minimal cerebral dysfunction. *Develop.
Med. Child Neurol.*, **8**, 71.

Karpeti G., Eisen A.H., Andermann F., Bacal H.L. & Robb P. (1965)
Ataxia telangiectasia. *Am. J. Dis. Child.*, **110**, 51.

Knobloch H. & Pasamanick B. (1959) Syndrome of minimal cerebral dam
age in infancy. *J. Am. Med. Ass.*, **170**, 1384.

Lucas A.R., Rodin E.A. & Simson C.B. (1965) Neurological assessment of
children with early school problems. *Develop. Med. Child Neurol.*, **7**, 145.

Ounsted C., Lindsay J. & Norman R. (1966) Biological Factors in Temporal
Lobe Epilepsy. *Clinics in Develop. Med. No. 22.* London, Heinemann.

Prechtl H.F.R. & Stemmer C.J. (1962) Choreiform syndrome in children.
Dev. Med. Child. Neurol., **4**, 119.

Paraesthesiae

Paraesthesiae are difficult to assess in children. The obvious cause of paraesthesiae in the legs is sitting with the legs crossed, or pressure of the edge of a chair against the back of the thigh.

Paraesthesiae may be one of the premonitory symptoms of *migraine* or a feature of *temporal lobe epilepsy*.

Overventilation as a result of hysteria or sulthiame may lead to paraesthesiae in the hands.

The symptom may be due to *drugs*—acetazolamide, amitriptyline, colistin, kanamycin, nalidixic acid, nitrofurantoin, piperazine, polymyxin, streptomycin, sulthiame, trimethoprim, thiobendazole or vincristine. Ergotamine may cause tingling, numbness and chilling of the extremities.

Undue excitement

This may be due to *hypoglycaemia*. It may also be caused by a variety of *drugs*, notably acetazolamide, antihistamines, chlordiazepoxide, diazepam, mepacrine, nitrofurantoin, nortryptiline, phenobarbitone and alcohol or poisons.

Undue irritability

The most likely cause of persistent undue irritability in a well child is *insecurity*, due probably to mismanagement—lack of real love, or excessive strictness and punishment. To some extent the irritability may be due to familial personality traits. It may be due to lassitude, boredom or anaemia.

179

When a school child habitually arrives home in a bad temper, the most likely cause is *hypoglycaemia*, responding rapidly to a meal. Otherwise he may have been bullied at school by a teacher or child.

A young baby's excessive irritability may be due to *phenylketonuria*. The infant with *coeliac disease* may vomit and become unduly irritable when given cereals.

Pink disease, due to mercury in teething powders or other substances should no longer be seen. It is characterised by pinkness of the hands and feet, excessive sweating, constant crying and photophobia.

Drugs are a most important cause of excessive irritability, and the worst offender is phenobarbitone. This may have a paradoxical effect of causing insomnia and irritability, particularly in mentally subnormal children. Primidone, which breaks down into a barbiturate, may have a similar action. Other drugs which may cause the symptoms include acetazolamide, aminophylline, amphetamine, antihistamines, ephedrine, fenfluramine (on withdrawal), imipramine, methimazole, sulthiame, thyroxin and troxidone.

Cyclopentolate, cycloserine, ethionamide, hyoscine and fenfluramine may give rise to a psychotic reaction and irritability.

In the case of a newborn infant, the *narcotic withdrawal syndrome* must be remembered if the mother is a drug addict.

Any illness, such as a *urinary tract infection*, may cause undue irritability.

Confusion and hallucinations

A short lasting confusional state may be a symptom of *migraine*, at the beginning of an attack. The child may have partial aphasia for a few minutes, and sometimes other neurological symptoms. The development of the headache helps to establish the diagnosis.

Temporal lobe epilepsy may be manifested by a confusional state or by abnormal behaviour of various kinds.

Hypoglycaemia commonly causes a confusional state.

Heat stroke or *dehydration* may be a cause.

Various *drugs*, in particular alcohol, amphetamine, antihistamines, cyclopentolate, diazepam, digoxin, ethionamide, ethosuccimide, fenfluramine, griseofulvin, hyoscine, indomethacin, mepacrine, monoamine, oxidase inhibitors, nitrofurantoin, phenytoin, piperazine, primidone and sulthiame, may be responsible.

Hallucinations may be a feature of *temporal lobe epilepsy*. They may be due to solvent sniffing, cannabis, LSD and various poisons.

Involuntary movement

The main causes of involuntary movements in children can be summarised as follows:

Moro and startle reflexes in the first three months
Sudden jerks in the young infant, mostly in sleep
Jaw trembling in the young baby
Jittery movements in the newborn, sometimes associated with tetany
     or hypoglycaemia
Hiccoughs
Tetany
Tics
Overactivity
Convulsions
Chorea
Tremors
Athetosis
Attacks of opisthotonos
Tetanus

Other causes are rare. They include the following:

Spasmus nutans
Spasmodic torticollis
Huntington's chorea
Dystonia musculorum deformans (torsion spasm)
Sequelae of encephalitis or meningitis

Subacute sclerosing panencephalitis and other degenerative diseases
    of the nervous system
Hepatolenticular degeneration
Lesch–Nyhan syndrome (see p. 185).
Drugs

All normal infants exhibit the *Moro* and *startle reflexes* in the
first three months. They are often excessive in infants suffering
from cerebral irritability. The Moro reflex consists of a sudden abduction of the arms at the shoulder with flexion at the elbow and
opening of the hands, followed by the hands coming together again.
It is due probably to vestibular reflexes set up by movement of the
neck, and is seen especially when the child is suddenly moved. The
startle reflex occurs as a result of a loud noise; it is somewhat different from the Moro reflex.

All normal children when asleep in the first few weeks have
sudden jerky movements resembling the startle reflex. Such movements in an infant who is awake may signify a convulsion. Many
newborn infants show a rapid jittering movement of the limbs. This
occurs in association with tetany or hypoglycaemia and in babies of
diabetic mothers.

All normal young infants show frequent *jaw trembling*.

Hiccoughs are normal in young infants after a feed. After infancy
they may be due to ethosuccimide or to a subphrenic abscess. Epidemic hiccough may be due to encephalitis, but more often hiccough,
lasting one to seven days followed by full recovery, follows a
respiratory infection.

For attacks of opisthotonos, see p. 184.

In the newborn period *tetany* is common. The clinical picture is
indistinguishable from that of other fits. It is only in the older child
that tetany, then rare, can be distinguished from fits by the typical
carpopedal spasm.

Tics are extremely common in children. They usually consist of
blinking the eyes, twitching the face, inappropriate mouth opening
('gaping'), shrugging the shoulders, sniffing or clucking the tongue.
They are usually single (i.e. one of the above), but may be multiple
and complex, and therefore readily confused with chorea. They are
more common in boys than in girls. The onset is more often at

about the age of seven years than at other ages, about 90 per cent beginning before the age of ten. They frequently disappear at puberty, but some persist throughout life. One tic usually lasts several months. Tics are brought on in the majority of cases by home conflicts and other causes of insecurity. The cause cannot be found in all cases.

Tics are commonly confused with *chorea*. The essential distinguishing feature is the fact that in a tic the same movement is constantly repeated; in chorea one never knows which movement is going to occur next. It is not by any means easy, however, to distinguish a complex tic from chorea of mild degree. In chorea one sees the characteristic hand posture when the child is asked to hold the hands out pronated. Severe chorea cannot be confused with tics because of the many other obvious features; but mild chorea may closely resemble tics.

I have often had children referred to me with the diagnosis of chorea, when the true diagnosis was mere *overactivity*. They did not show the varied uncoordinated movements of chorea. *Convulsions* are discussed on p. 186. There may be twitching of a hemiplegic limb without loss of consciousness.

Spasmus nutans is a peculiar condition seen in infants aged usually three to about 24 months, in which there are rhythmical jerky movements of the neck, in the lateral or horizontal direction, but sometimes vertical, ceasing when the child concentrates on an object. The child often has a characteristic way of looking at objects out of his eye corners and may tilt his head to one side. The movements disappear in sleep. Nystagmus is usually present and is often more marked on one side than the other. It is increased by holding the head still. It disappears spontaneously by the age of three or four.

Spasmodic torticollis is related to tics and is probably psychogenic in origin. The child or adult shows sudden single lateral movements of the neck. The head is often held tilted to one side.

Huntington's chorea is a rare dominant degenerative disease of the nervous system, usually appearing after childhood, but sometimes showing itself as early as six. There is first an emotional change, followed by chorea and then dementia and convulsions, ending in death.

Dystonia musculorum deformans (torsion spasm) begins between the age of five and ten, with hypertonus of the calf muscles, leading to inversion and adduction of the foot, with a typical deformity. Later there is a fixed flexion and adduction of the hip, with lordosis and torticollis and painful involuntary movements.

Parkinsonian-like movements may result from *epidemic encephalitis* or from certain forms of *meningitis*. They may also be a side effect of cephalosporins. Tremors or Parkinsonism may be caused by amitriptyline, amphetamine, imipramine, phenytoin or the phenothiazines. Tremor in the hands is common in children, especially in mentally subnormal ones. The tremor is seen particularly on fine manipulation, as on building a tower of cubes.

Subacute sclerosing panencephalitis is a rare condition beginning with ordinary fits, but leading to sudden rhythmical convulsive movements, dementia and death in a few weeks. The electroencephalogram shows characteristic tracings. It may sometimes be an unusual response to the measles virus or other infection.

Hepatolenticular degeneration is a rare recessive metabolic condition showing itself usually in later childhood. The symptoms are those of a basal ganglion lesion, with difficulty in speech and swallowing, a fixed rigid face, with involuntary movements, dysarthria, tremor, inappropriate laughter, muscle rigidity, pericorneal pigmentation, tremor and dementia, with cirrhosis of the liver. The diagnosis may be confirmed by estimation of the serum caeruloplasmin.

Tetanus causes spasms which may be confused with epileptic fits. The excessive muscle tone and therefore stiffness in between the convulsive movements, together with the history of trauma, should point to the diagnosis.

Opisthotonos. Opisthotonos in a newborn baby has to be distinguished from the posture assumed by a baby who was delivered with a *face presentation*. Such babies are not hypertonic and therefore do not have opisthotonos. In developing countries in which undesirable substances are placed on the newborn's umbilicus, tetanus is a common cause.

Opisthotonos is a feature of *hypertonia*, and attacks of it may be an early sign of *athetosis*, before athetoid movements appear. The condition may result from *meningitis* which has been improperly treated or which has not responded well to treatment. It may result from *injury to the neck*. It is often seen in infants with a *vascular*

ing. It may result from *retropharyngeal abscess or lymphadenitis.*
It may be due to *drugs,* especially the phenothiazines, or to poison,
such as methaqualone (Mandrax). Opisthotonos due to drugs may
be associated with torsion spasms or Parkinsonism.

Attacks of opisthotonos may occur in the *Lesch-Nyhan syndrome*
of hyperuricaemia, self mutilation, dystonic movements or athetosis,
and mental defect, a rare condition mostly confined to boys.

References

HOEFNAGEL D. & BIERY B. (1968) Spasmus Nutans. *Develop. Med. Child Neurol.,* **10,** 32.
TORUP E. (1962) A follow-up study of children with tics. *Acta Paediat. Uppsala,* **51,** 261.

Convulsions

Convulsions are common in children. About six to seven per cent
of all children have one or more convulsions. They are particularly
common in children with mental deficiency or cerebral palsy. In
my experience about 20 per cent of mentally defective children have
fits, with the exception of mongols, of whom only about one per
cent have convulsions. The overall incidence of convulsions in
cerebral palsy is about 35 per cent. Fits occur in almost 50 per cent
of children with spastic hemiplegia, in perhaps 40 per cent of children with spastic quadriplegia, but in a smaller proportion of those
with spastic diplegia. In athetoids they occur in about ten per cent,
and they rarely occur in those with congenital ataxia. There are
scores of possible causes of fits, and because in some of these conditions early diagnosis is vital, it is wrong for a family doctor to guess
at the diagnosis, pay little attention to the fits and therefore fail
to obtain the opinion of a specialist, who may feel that certain
special investigations should be carried out. Failure to seek the help

of a specialist may under some circumstances cause the child to become mentally defective, whereas with treatment he would have been normal. Failure to take fits seriously may in other cases directly lead to a child's death. Apart from this, convulsions cause great distress to parents, and for various reasons lead to serious emotional difficulties in children. *When an infant or child has a convulsion it is essential that every step should be taken to establish the correct diagnosis in order that the appropriate treatment can be given. Convulsions are not due to teething. One has seen many disasters which have resulted from ascribing convulsions to this cause.*

A convulsion is the end result of any one of a very wide variety of causes. From the nature of the convulsions one can rarely make a diagnosis of the cause, because most convulsions in children look alike, with the exception of *petit mal* and *infantile spasms*.

The common causes vary with the child's age. In a newborn baby the commonest causes of a convulsion are a brain defect or injury (as by anoxia), hypoglycaemia or hypocalcaemia. In some countries tetanus is a common cause. Febrile convulsions and epilepsy are rarely found in the first six months.

From six months to five years the commonest diagnosis will be a febrile convulsion, though breath-holding fits are not uncommon. After the age of two or three, epileptic fits become common, and after the age of five the usual diagnosis will be epilepsy.

The subject will now be discussed under the headings of the three age periods.

The newborn period

A convulsion in a newborn baby rarely presents as an obvious major fit. It commonly presents as mere twitching of limb or limbs. The twitching may migrate from one limb or part of the body to another. Examination of such a baby may show that there is conjugate deviation of the eyes and that he is stiff. Convulsive movements have to be distinguished from the normal sudden jerks on awakening, and from the agitation and tremulousness shown by a baby when hungry. Clonic movements of a limb cannot be stopped by flexing the limb, whilst jittering tremulous movements can. (Brown *et al.*, 1972.) There is no doubt that many convulsions masquerade as cyanotic attacks (p. 124). In other words, what is thought to be a cyanotic attack is in fact the end result of a convulsion.

The main causes to consider are as follows:

Tetany
Hypomagnesaemia
Hypoglycaemia
Brain defect or injury:
  Congenital defects
  Anoxia
  Cerebral oedema
  Subdural effusion, cerebal haemorrhage
Fructosaemia, galactosaemia, lactose intolerance
Serum sodium high
Infection, tetanus
Pyridoxine dependency
Maple syrup urine disease; homocystinuria
Kernicterus
Narcotic withdrawal syndrome
Effect of drugs

In Britain the three main causes of neonatal convulsions are brain defect or injury, hypoglycaemia and hypocalcaemia. There are many other but less frequent causes.

Brain defect or injury. These include serious congenital brain defects, anoxia before or during birth, cerebral oedema, subdural haematoma or other intracranial haemorrhage. Nothing can be done about the congenital brain defect or about the effects of anoxia, but cerebral oedema may be relieved by measures in hospital and increased intracranial pressure from a cerebral haemorrhage may occasionally be relieved by lumbar puncture even though this procedure has its risks. Subdural haematoma is an unusual cause of fits in the newborn baby. Convulsions on the first day are more likely to be due to anoxia; on the second or third day they are more likely to be due to cerebral haemorrhage.

If there is a serious brain defect, the cranial circumference may be unusually small, but it is not always so. If there is cerebral oedema or a subdural effusion, the fontanelle is likely to be bulging and the sutures may be widely separated. There may be retinal haemorrhages, but such haemorrhages are often found in normal babies. In most full-term infants the symptoms of cerebral haemorrhage commonly develop on about the third day, the infant having been previously well. The child suddenly has cyanotic attacks or convulsions, may vomit and go off his food. There may be bulging of the fontanelle. He may develop atelectasis and so develop respiratory symptoms which mask the real cause, a cerebral haemorrhage.

Neonatal hypoglycaemia. Neonatal hypoglycaemia occurs particularly in babies who are small in relation to the duration of gestation, in babies of toxaemic mothers, in boys rather than in girls, in the smaller of twins and in babies of diabetic mothers. It follows birth injury or cold injury, and may be associated with the respiratory distress syndrome, kernicterus, Beckwith's syndrome (umbilical hernia with macroglossia and hypoglycaemia), adrenocortical hyperplasia, infections and glycogenoses. The symptoms begin a few hours after birth in most babies, but a few develop them up to five or six days later. They consist of twitches, cyanotic attacks and convulsions. The diagnosis can be made with certainty only by estimating the blood glucose. It is important to establish the diagnosis promptly in order that appropriate treatment can be given.

A baby may vomit and have a fit when first given milk, as a result of *lactose intolerance*, *fructosaemia*, or *galactosaemia*.

Neonatal tetany. This is due largely to the inability of the newborn baby to handle the high phosphorus content of cow's milk. It is also related to physiological hypocalcaemia, which occurs particularly between the third and the fifth or sixth days. It may occur when the mother has suffered from hyperparathyroidism or diabetes in pregnancy. There may be associated hypomagnesaemia. The symptoms are convulsions which are indistinguishable from other convulsions. The typical carpopedal spasm of tetany in older children is rarely seen. A positive Chvosek's sign does not establish the diagnosis because it occurs in normal babies. It is important that the correct diagnosis should be made in order that treatment can be given. The prognosis is better for this condition than it is for other causes of convulsions in the newborn period.

Fits in the newborn period can also be due to an abnormally *low or high level of the serum sodium*. They may also be due to the mother having taken large quantities of pyridoxine in pregnancy. Pyridoxine dependency is a rare cause of fits in the newborn.

Infections. Any severe infection may cause convulsions in the newborn period. Infections include septicaemia and pyogenic meningitis. It is important to remember that there is usually neither neck stiffness nor a positive Kernig's sign in neonatal meningitis, and there may be no bulging of the fontanelle. The baby is just ill and no good reason can be found for it. It is easy to miss the diagnosis of an E. coli or similar meningitis in the newborn period, and the result is disastrous—death or hydrocephalus. In the same way septicaemia can readily be missed. A low-grade one will show itself only by loss of appetite and perhaps a low-grade anaemia, but in severe cases there may be convulsions, haemorrhages, jaundice and vomiting. The sticky umbilicus is a common source of infection.

Other infections, not so serious, may cause convulsions. They include otitis media and pneumonia. Rare infections include toxoplasmosis, generalised herpes and cytomegalovirus infection.

Neonatal tetanus is almost unknown in the United Kingdom, but common in certain countries abroad in which goat dung, cow dung, mud or other undesirable materials are applied to the umbilicus at birth. The first symptom is usually difficulty in sucking at the age of five or six days followed by stiffness of the jaw and generalised spasticity. Twitchings develop and spasms occur spontaneously or in response to stimulation. The child lies stiffly with flexed extremities or opisthotonos, with a risus sardonicus, stiff jaws, or a stiff upper lip on feeding, and short spasms accompanied by little snorts or grunts (Marshall, 1968).

Other metabolic conditions causing convulsions in the young baby are maple syrup urine disease, homocystinuria and hypersarcosinaemia.

Kernicterus commonly presents at the age of five to nine days in infants with hyperbilirubinaemia, as a result of haemolytic disease or prematurity. Fits may be a feature.

The narcotic withdrawal syndrome has been described in the United States. When the mother is a morphine or heroin addict the baby at birth will suffer the symptoms of withdrawal—extreme irritability, convulsions and excessive salivation.

Drugs given for the treatment of neonatal asphyxia, such as nikethamide or ethamivan, may cause convulsions if only a small overdose is given.

Convulsions in infants after the newborn period

The following conditions should be considered:

Febrile convulsions
Breath-holding attacks
Brain defects
   Subdural effusion
   Head injury
Epilepsy including infantile spasms
Sequelae of immunisation
Intracranial infections
Metabolic conditions
   Hypoglycaemia, tetany, phenylketonuria, glycinaemia, pyridoxine dependency, maple syrup urine disease, homocystinuria, citrullinuria, argininosuccinicaciduria.
Dehydration and its repair
Infections (other than those causing febrile convulsions)
Poisons
Sickle cell anaemia
The haemolytic uraemic syndrome (pp. 48, 86)
Acute infantile hemiplegia
Acute nephritis

After the first weeks of life and up to the age of four or five years the commonest cause of fits is the so-called *febrile convulsion*. This condition is the source of much confusion. It is important to distinguish it from epilepsy because the treatment and the prognosis are different. The following are the criteria necessary for making the diagnosis:

(1) Febrile convulsions are definitely unusual before the age of six months, and they should not be diagnosed after the age of five years. The peak age incidence is eighteen months.

(2) They only occur with a rapid rise of temperature, and there must be a history of the child having been off colour and probably off his food for a few hours before the fit occurred.

(3) Fits occurring more than 12 hours after the onset of an illness are almost certainly not febrile convulsions, unless there is a complication such as otitis media developing after a sore throat.

(4) The fits should not last more than ten minutes.

(5) They should be general and not focal.

(6) There must be no history of fits without a precipitating infection.

(7) There should be only one fit with the rapid rise of temperature. A series of fits would make the diagnosis unlikely.

(8) There must not be residual weakness of a limb (Todd's paralysis) after a fit.

(9) The EEG between fits is normal.

There are some important difficulties with regard to the diagnosis. Firstly, fever may precipitate fits in epileptics. Hence the criteria above must be satisfied. In particular there must be no history of fits in between the 'febrile convulsions'. Secondly, any severe convulsion may cause a rise of temperature. Hence the finding of an elevated temperature following a fit does not prove that an infection caused the fit.

If a child has an infection which caused both an elevation of temperature and a fit, the temperature may have dropped in transit to the hospital. Hence the finding of definite infection together with the appropriate history may be more important for the diagnosis than the finding of an elevated temperature.

A family history of febrile convulsions is commonly obtained, but a family history of definite epilepsy would arouse doubts about the diagnosis of febrile fits.

Breath-holding convulsions may occur at any age between about six months and five years. The usual age of onset is six to eighteen months. The child when thwarted or hurt may cry, hold his breath in expiration, or cry, 'Till all the air has gone out of his lungs', as a parent said. The child rapidly becomes blue, and if he holds the breath for a further ten or fifteen seconds, he becomes limp. If he holds the breath for a further ten or fifteen seconds, he will have a major convulsion indistinguishable from epilepsy. It is important to note the exact sequence of events, for this sequence helps one to distinguish the attacks from epileptic fits. In a typical epileptic fit the child has a sudden convulsion, becoming stiff first, then twitches and becomes blue. There is no aura and no preceding stimulus (pain or thwarting). If there is a cry it is synchronous with the tonic phase; this is followed by the clonic phase. Cyanosis occurs late in the epileptic fit, not at the beginning, as it does in a breath-holding attack. A fit following anger or fright is unlikely to be epilepsy.

Toronto neurologists have described a pallid type of breath-holding attack usually following pain; in it there is rapid loss of consciousness with pallor but without preceding cyanosis. In both types there is commonly a family history of similar fits.

Many make the mistake of thinking that breath-holding attacks are merely a behaviour problem, occurring only when the child cannot get his own way. In fact they commonly occur when the child has a fall or other injury. It has been suggested that there is some association with hypochromic anaemia.

Anti-epileptic drugs do not affect the frequency of the attacks—a useful therapeutic test when one is in doubt. The EEG is normal and no other investigation is necessary.

Brain defects. Congenital brain defects, such as cerebral agenesis or porencephalic cysts, are an important cause of fits in the older baby. In a high proportion of these there will be associated mental subnormality or neurological signs suggesting cerebral palsy. Fits are an unusual complication of congenital hydrocephalus. In the first year of life and perhaps in the first two years brain defects are a more common cause of fits than epilepsy.

Subdural effusion and head injury. Convulsions occur as a result of a serious head injury, but they also occur as a result of subdural effusion or haematoma which often presents without any definite evidence of injury. It is well known that in child abuse all possibility of it being anything but accidental is stoutly denied. All small children receive some bumps on the head in falls, and it seems that a subdural effusion may result from an apparently minor injury or from violent shaking. The presenting symptom is a convulsion or a too rapidly enlarging head. The diagnosis is made by ophthalmoscopic finding of retinal haemorrhages, by transillumination of the skull and by subdural tap.

Epilepsy may occur in infancy, but it should be regarded as being probably secondary to some cause such as a brain defect or metabolic condition.

Infantile spasms. The so-called infantile spasms have also been termed 'Salaam spasms', 'myoclonic seizures' and 'hypsarrhythmic attacks'. They consist of sudden rapid flexion of the trunk, lasting a fraction of a second. The subject has been fully reviewed by Jeavons and Bower (1964). In 70 per cent of cases the attacks begin during the first six months, particularly at about four to six months of age. They usually cease by the age of eighteen months, but are commonly replaced by major convulsions. They are not examples of *petit mal* epilepsy, with which they are commonly confused. The attacks may result from a wide variety of causes—such as gross brain defects and damage, subdural haematoma, phenylketonuria, severe hypoglycaemia, tuberous sclerosis, the Sturge-Weber syndrome (facial portwine stain with mental deficiency, cerebral palsy and fits), Tay-Sach's disease, congenital syphilis and other causes. The condition is not a specific entity. In 16 of the 157 cases described by Jeavons and Bower the attacks followed within a week of triple immunisation. It is the end result of a wide variety of pathological processes, though in 97 per cent the EEG is characteristic—showing the so-called 'hypsarrhythmia'—sudden high peaks of electrical activity.

Immunisation. If an infant has a convulsion a few hours after the triple immunisation, no further injection of the triple vaccine should be given, though it is safe to continue immunisation against tetanus by giving tetanus toxoid. The convulsion may be due to encephalitis, but it may be a mere febrile convulsion following a rapid rise of temperature resulting from the injection. As one cannot be sure what has caused the fit, unless there are other signs of encephalitis, one must not take the risk of giving more triple vaccine.

Intracranial infections. Pyogenic meningitis may cause convulsions and it is easy to make a mistaken diagnosis of a febrile convulsion when in fact the child has meningitis. Even if there is an obvious infection, such as otitis media, pyogenic meningitis cannot be excluded in an infant or young child without a lumbar puncture, because in the infant there is not always neck stiffness. For this reason *cerebrospinal fluid examination should always be carried out when a child has what is thought to be a febrile fit*. I saw a small child who had a fit and who on examination was found to have an upper lobe pneumonia. There was no neck stiffness or other sign of meningism. On lumbar puncture it was found that he had pneumococcal meningitis.

Poliomyelitis and other forms of *encephalitis* may be accompanied by a convulsion at the onset. It will be remembered that *paroxysmal vertigo* can be confused with epilepsy.

Hypoglycaemia. It is important to remember that convulsions may be due to hypoglycaemia, other than that due to insulin over-dosage. It is of vital importance that the diagnosis should be established, because recurrent hypoglycaemic attacks with convulsions cause irreparable brain damage. The fit is commonly preceded by weakness, pallor and sweating.

Hypoglycaemia may be due to hyperplasia or tumour of the islets of Langerhans, hypopituitarism, adrenocortical insufficiency, glycogenoses, hepatic disease or carbohydrate intolerance. With regard to the latter, an example is fructose intolerance, in which the child has hypoglycaemic symptoms such as vomiting, malaise and tremors on eating sweats. Investigation for these conditions is laborious and should be carried out in hospital. It will include glucagon and adrenalin tolerance tests and tests of liver, pituitary and adrenal function.

Tetany. Tetany after the newborn period is due to a variety of causes, including rickets, steatorrhoea, alkalosis, hypoparathyroidism or damage to the parathyroid glands following thyroidectomy for thyrotoxicosis. In older children hysterical overventilation may cause tetany. Tetany due to rickets occurs especially between the age of four months and three years. The clinical diagnosis of rickets is made by the thickened epiphyses of the wrist and the enlarged costochondral junctions. There is commonly some anaemia and hypotonia. The diagnosis can only be suspected on clinical grounds, but it must be confirmed by x-ray of the wrist or costochondral junctions and the serum alkaline phosphatase. Owing to the relative frequency of resistant rickets in Britain, one must not be misled by the history that adequate doses of Vitamin D have been given, though tetany in resistant rickets is rare.

Fits due to tetany are commonly indistinguishable from other major convulsions. Occasionally, however, one may see the typical limb posture of tetany—the thumb drawn into the palm of the hand, the hands abducted with the wrists flexed, the fingers flexed at the metacarpo-phalangeal joints and extended at the distal joints.

Dehydration following gastroenteritis and sometimes respiratory tract infections may be accompanied by convulsions. The causes are varied, and include electrolyte disturbances such as hyponatraemia, hypernatraemia and hypocalcaemia; over-rapid hydration; hydraemia as a result of overhydration; hyperthermia; and cerebral thrombosis. It may result from giving too much fluid without sufficient sodium or from hydrating too rapidly.

Other metabolic conditions listed are diagnosed by paper chromatography and other means. Phenylketonuria is best diagnosed in the newborn period by the Guthrie test, which depends on the serum phenylalanine in heel-prick blood.

Infections—such as postinfectious encephalomyelitis associated with the common infectious diseases, whooping cough and toxoplasmosis are causes of fits. Post infectious encephalomyelitis commonly follows an acute infectious disease, but may occasionally precede the rash in the case of the exanthems or the parotid swelling in the case of mumps. Occasionally the encephalitic symptoms occur without the appearance of the rash or the mumps, the diagnosis being made by virological means.

Poisons. The possibility of poisoning should always be borne in mind when a child has an obscure illness. Numerous poisons and drugs may cause convulsions; they include amitriptyline, antihistamines, camphor, chlorpromazine, corticosteroids, dicophane, insulin overdosage, lead, phenothiazine, strychnine.

The so-called *acute infantile hemiplegia* is the result of a variety of conditions, such as infections, injury, immunisation, congenital heart disease, disseminated lupus erythematosus, periarteritis, sickle cell anaemia, polycythaemia, thrombocytopenic purpura and dehydration. The child has a major and often protracted convulsion followed by coma, and is then found to have a hemiplegia with mental subnormality.

Convulsions after infancy

Febrile convulsions (until the age of five)
Epilepsy

Breath-holding attacks (until the age of five)
Faints
Hysteria; overventilation tetany
Brain diseases
Head injury
Intracranial infections
Encephalitis
Whooping cough
Hypoglycaemia
Metabolic conditions, including dehydration and insulin overdosage
Nephritis and hypertension
Poison
Drugs
Haemolytic uraemic syndrome (pp. 48, 86)

Febrile convulsions and breath-holding attacks have virtually ceased by the age of five, but are common before then, especially between the age of one and three or four years.

Many of the conditions already mentioned must be considered in the older child. The most common cause of fits after the fifth year is *epilepsy*. Many children are thought to have *petit mal* when in fact they have infantile spasms or more often *grand mal*. The distinction is of great importance in the case of *petit mal* and *grand mal*, for the treatment of the two conditions is different. The drug of choice for *petit mal* is ethosuccimide, while that for *grand mal* is phenobarbitone or phenytoin, neither of which is helpful in treating *petit mal*.

Petit mal consists of brief lapses of consciousness, lasting up to 20 seconds, without a preceding aura, without convulsive movements and not followed by sleep. The attacks are commonly called 'dizzy spells' or 'fainting turns'. The child may stop, stand and stare. There may be flickering of the eyelids and a momentary upward deviation of the eyes, but there is no twitching of the limbs. Not more than five per cent of affected children fall in an attack. There is no change in colour. The child may drop an object held in the hand and may wet himself. The attacks can almost always be precipitated by forced overventilation.

Petit mal is distinguished from infantile spasms by the following features:

(1) The age incidence. Infantile spasms occur mainly at four to six months and cease by three. *Petit mal* is rare before three, occurs predominantly between the age of four and eight years, usually ceasing by puberty (when it may be replaced by *grand mal*).

(2) The duration of the attacks. The duration of *petit mal* is longer than that of infantile spasms, which consist of a sudden jack-knife flexion lasting a fraction of a second.

(3) Infantile spasms are almost always associated with mental deficiency, while in 95 per cent of children with *petit mal* the IQ is normal.

(4) The EEG is different. The EEG in infantile spasms shows sudden peaks of electrical discharge: that of *petit mal* shows three per second spike and wave activity.

Petit mal is distinguished from *grand mal* by the following points:

(1) The rarity of *petit mal*. *Petit mal* is a relatively rare form of fit in children. It occurred in two to three per cent of 15,102 epileptics seen at the Johns Hopkins Hospital at Baltimore.

(2) The nature of the fit. Convulsive twitching in a limb suggests *grand mal*. A fall usually signifies *grand mal*. Stiffness in an attack signifies *grand mal*. A change of colour is against the diagnosis of *petit mal*.

(3) The duration of the fit. *Grand mal* can be momentary, but it usually lasts longer. A *petit mal* attack lasts not more than 20 seconds.

(4) *Petit mal* attacks can usually be precipitated by overventilation. The child is instructed to blow 100 times a piece of paper 12 inches away.

(5) *Grand mal* attacks are commonly followed by sleep and sometimes by vomiting. This does not apply to *petit mal*.

(6) The EEG is different. The EEG is abnormal in children with *petit mal*, showing the three per second spike and wave activity. It is often normal in children with *grand mal*.

There are many different kinds of epileptic fit. In *temporal lobe epilepsy* there may be aurae consisting of hallucinations of smell, taste, sight or hearing. There may also be feelings of fear or abdominal pain. Chewing and odd movements may occur. There may be sudden tachycardia, blanching followed by blushing, paroxysmal confusion, meaningless words, senseless laughter, delusions or hallucinations, and catastrophic rage, with violent unexplained outbursts of temper. It may follow anoxia, pyogenic meningitis, encephalitis, head injury, a prolonged fit of any cause, Schildler's disease, tuberous sclerosis or phenylketonuria (Ounsted, 1966).

Psychomotor epilepsy may show itself by sudden unexplained temper tantrums. These should be considered when an epileptic child has unexplained outbursts of temper and screaming. Epileptic automatism occurs in children—leading to sudden irrational acts, such as walking fully clothed into a lake.

By no means all epileptic children have tonic and clonic phases in a fit. Some have unexplained falls and are limp when picked up, without twitching.

A sudden instantaneous onset of headache or of abdominal pain, lasting a few minutes only and followed by sleep may be a manifestation of epilepsy.

It can be difficult to distinguish *faints* from fits. Faints are definitely rare in a young child, but from early puberty to adolescence they are common. A faint usually occurs on change of posture or on prolonged standing (as in school prayers), while a fit may occur at any time (particularly on awakening or on going to sleep). If a mother tells me that her child 'faints' when sitting in a chair I would certainly say that her diagnosis was incorrect, an epileptic fit being far more likely. Likewise if a child suddenly 'faints' when playing it is far more likely to be an epileptic fit. Loss of colour or limpness can occur with either faint or fit. Convulsive movements can occasionally occur during a faint, though it is an infrequent occurrence: they do not definitely point to the diagnosis of epilepsy. An EEG may help in the diagnosis, but one must remember that the EEG is normal in many cases of *grand mal* epilepsy, and a fit resembling a faint would be *grand mal*, not *petit mal*.

Hysteria and hysterical overventilation tetany are unusual in children. They are confined to older children—after the age of six or seven years. The hysterical fit is not difficult to distinguish from epilepsy, but when a mother describes an attack of hysterical over-ventilation tetany it is easy to make a wrong diagnosis. The history of overventilation followed by tingling in the extremities and stiff-ness of the hands and feet (perhaps with a description of carpopedal spasm), should make one think of tetany.

Epilepsy can closely simulate attacks of *paroxysmal vertigo* (p. 170).

Various neurodermatoses, such as *tuberous sclerosis* and the *Sturge-Weber syndrome* (with a portwine stain on the face) are associated with fits. In the case of tuberous sclerosis, the mother may have the typical facial lesions, which will point to the diag-nosis; children do not usually have the facial lesions in the first five years or so.

It has already been stated that fits are common in severely defec-tive children other than mongols. They are common in degenerative diseases of the nervous system.

A severe head injury, a cerebral abscess or a subdural effusion may be followed in months or years by convulsions. In some ten per cent or more of children in whom convulsions follow these con-ditions, the first fit may not occur until ten years or more after the damage to the brain was inflicted.

Intracranial infections, including meningitis and encephalitis, con-tinue to be important causes of fits. Post-infectious encephalo-myelitis following the common infectious diseases is also important.

Metabolic conditions are important causes of fits. They include in particular hypoglycaemia, whether spontaneous or the result of insulin overdosage, and the effects of dehydration and repair. The symptoms of ketotic hypoglycaemia commonly begin after the first birthday, especially in low birth weight babies who have remained small and thin. The symptoms may be drowsiness in the morning before eating or at other times of food deprivation. The diagnosis is established in hospital.

Convulsions are an important complication of *acute nephritis,* when there is associated hypertension. A child with acute nephritis should be referred to hospital in order that appropriate treatment can be given to prevent fits if the blood pressure is dangerously high. It should be noted that rarely acute nephritis may occur without albuminaria.

Poisons, especially lead, are important causes of fits. Other poisons include amphetamines, carbon tetrachloride, dicophane, lead, mercury, monoamine oxidase inhibitors, pyrethrum, rotenone and strychnine.

Drugs which cause fits include acetazolamide, aminophylline, amitriptyline, antihistamines, carbamazepine, chlorpromazine, corticosteroids, cycloserine, imipramine, isoniazid, nalidixic acid and the phenothiazines.

References

BROWN J.K., COCKBURN F. & FORFAR J.O. (1972) Clinical and chemical correlations in convulsions in the newborn. *Lancet, 1*, 135.

CARTER S. & GOLD A. (1967) Acute Infantile Hemiplegia. *Pediat. Clinics. N. Am.*, **14**, 851.

CHAO D., SEXTON J.A. & PARDO L. (1962) Temporal lobe epilepsy in children. *J. Pediat.*, **60**, 686.

FREEMAN J.M. (1970) Neonatal seizures—diagnosis and management. *J. Pediat.*, **77**. 710.

GAUK E.W., KIDD L. & PRICHARD J.S. (1963) Mechanism of seizures associated with breath-holding spells. *New Engl. J. Med.*, **268**, 1436.

HOYER J.R., MICHAEL A.F., FISH A.J. & GOOD R.A. (1967) Acute post-streptococcal glomerulonephritis presenting as hypertensive encephalopathy with minimal urinary abnormalities. *Pediatrics*, **39**, 412.

JEAVONS P.M. & BOWER B.D. (1964) Infantile spasms. *Developmental Clinics, No. 15*. London, Heinemann.

LENNOX M.A. (1949) Febrile Convulsions in Childhood. *Am. J. Dis. Child.*, **78**, 868.

LENNOX W.G. (1960) *Epilepsy and related disorders*. Boston, Little Brown & Co.

LOMBROSO C.T. & LERMAN P. (1967) Breath-holding spells (cynotic and pallid infantile syncope). *Pediatrics*, **39**, 563.

MARSHALL F. (1968) Tetanus of the newborn. *Adv. in Pediatrics*. Vol. 15. Year Book Publishing Co.

OUNSTED C., LINDSAY J. & NORMAN R. (1966) Biological factors in temporal lobe epilepsy. *Clinics in Develop. Med. No. 22*. London, Heinemann.

PAINE R. (1968) Characteristics of fits in the newborn period. *Clinics in Develop. Med. No. 27*, **70**. London, Heinemann.

ROSE A.L. & LOMBROSO C.T. (1970) Neonatal seizure states. *Pediatrics*, **45**, 404.

Coma

When a child is referred to one because of coma, the first conditions to think about are as follows:

Diabetic coma
Hypoglycaemia, due to insulin overdosage
Effect of drugs and poisons
Head injury
Epilepsy
Meningitis or encephalitis
Cerebral haemorrhage, abscess or tumour, or other cause of increased intracranial pressure

Other causes include:

Other severe infections, such as meningococcal septicaemia
Liver failure—such as severe hepatitis or the sequel of cirrhosis
Kidney failure—uraemia
Sodium deficiency and dehydration: hypernatraemia
    Dehydration in association with an infection or excessive heat
    Addison's disease
Hysteria

In the case of *diabetes* and *insulin overdosage*, a history of diabetes is a great help to the diagnosis. The smell of acetone in the breath should suggest diabetic acidosis, and there may be sugar in the urine. A rare though important form of diabetic coma is the nonketotic hyperosmolar form with hyperglycaemia, dehydration, fits, mild or moderate diabetes, but without significant acidosis or ketosis.

Numerous *drugs* when taken in excess may cause coma. The most common one is a barbiturate. As stated elsewhere, the parents' statement that the child has not had access to drugs should not be taken to eliminate poisoning. When a known epileptic lapses into coma, one must always think of the possibility of barbiturate poisoning (deliberate or otherwise). Salicylate poisoning may also cause coma, and the phenistix test helps to diagnose this. Cyclopentolate (mydriatic) may cause delirium and coma. Other drugs or poisons which cause coma include alcohol, amphetamine, aminophylline, arsenic, carbon monoxide, iron, kerosene, lead, mushroom poisoning, organic phosphates, phenothiazines, piperazine, phenytoin, thallium.

The head should always be examined for evidence of *injury*, and the optic fundi should be examined for papilloedema or haemorrhages.

Coma may be due to *meningitis, encephalitis* or *cerebral haemorrhage, tumour* or *abscess*, and a lumbar puncture will be done in hospital unless there is papilloedema.

Infective hepatitis can be acute and lead to coma in a few hours. The Kussmaul breathing of *uraemia* should point to renal failure.

Severe dehydration can occur rapidly, particularly in infants or defective children, usually when they have a respiratory infection or gastroenteritis, and severe dehydration may cause a surprising degree of nitrogen retention and even coma.

Hysteria is a possible cause of coma in an older child.

Reference

Arieff A.I. & Carroll H.J. (1972) Nonketotic hyperosmolar coma with hyperglycaemia. *Medicine,* 51, 73.

Drowsiness

Undue drowsiness may be due merely to *fatigue* or *lack of sleep* if the child is otherwise well.

It may be due to any *serious illness*, including febrile conditions, meningitis, diabetic acidosis and uraemia.

A variety of *drugs* cause drowsiness. They include all the drugs used in the treatment of epilepsy, antihistamines, diphenoxylate, fenfluramine, indomethacin, meprobamate, methimazole, nalidixic acid, P.A.S., the phenothiazines and tranquillising drugs. *Poisons* should be considered.

Drowsiness may be due to dehydration including heatstroke and hypernatraemia. It may be due to hypernatraemia which has been caused by the baby's feeds being made up too concentrated. It is sometimes an early symptom of hypoglycaemia.

Reference

STERN G.M., JONES R.B. & FRASER A.C.L. (1972) Hyperosmolar dehydration in infancy due to faulty feeding. *Arch. Dis. Childh.*, **47**, 468.

Neck stiffness

Neck stiffness may be a symptom or sign of the utmost importance in childhood, in that it may point to meningitis. On the other hand it may be a trivial matter of no importance. The main causes are as follows:

Acute
  Meningism
  Meningitis and encephalitis
  Intracranial haemorrhage, abscess, tumour
  Neck injury
  Osteitis of cervical vertebrae
  The effects of lumbar puncture
  'Rheumatic stiff neck'
  Rheumatoid arthritis
  Inflamed cervical lymph nodes
  Retropharyngeal abscess or lymph nodes
  Drugs

Chronic
  Congenital abnormalities of the vertebrae
  Myositis ossificans
  Cerebral palsy of the spastic or rigid type
  Sternomastoid tumour (in the infant)
  Rheumatoid arthritis

The neck stiffness of *meningism* and meningitis consists of stiffness in flexing the neck, but not in lateral movement. Ideally the child should be in the sitting position when the test is carried out. The neck is fully extended and then flexed. Resistance may be felt throughout the movement of flexion or only in the terminal part of the movement, when the chin is almost touching the sternum. It is important to watch the child's face when testing for meningism, for if there is meningism there is almost always pain on flexing the neck. A wince of pain in the last part of the movement may be the only convincing sign of meningism. The pain is usually felt in the lumbar region, but is sometimes felt in the muscle at the back of the neck. The child with meningism may be unable to kiss his knees. When he sits up in bed he exhibits the tripod sign, placing both arms behind him so that he does not fall back owing to spasm of the glutei, erector spinae and hamstrings.

Meningism occurs in a variety of infections in childhood, such as pneumonia, pyelonephritis, otitis media, tonsillitis, infective hepatitis, mumps and typhoid fever. It occurs in many virus infections of the nervous system, such as poliomyelitis, encephalitis, the post-infectious encephalomyelitides and pyogenic meningitis. It also occurs after an intracranial haemorrhage or in the presence of a cerebral abscess or a tumour.

It is essential that a lumbar puncture should be performed as soon as meningism is found, because it is impossible otherwise to be sure that the child has not a pyogenic meningitis, requiring appropriate antibiotic treatment. It is disastrous either to wait and see how the child progresses or to prescribe an antibiotic. If that is done, it will be impossible subsequently to identify the organism so that the correct treatment can be given. For this reason, the child should be referred to a hospital so that a lumbar puncture can be performed and the appropriate examination of the cerebro-spinal fluid can be carried out.

Neck stiffness may result from an *injury to the neck*, such as a dislocation or fracture, or from *osteitis of the vertebrae.*

After a *lumbar puncture* there may be some pain on flexing the neck. This could be confused with meningism.

The so-called *'rheumatic stiff neck'* is a mysterious entity, at one time ascribed to sitting in a draught. Davies (1960) described an epidemic of painful stiff neck in 13 nurses. He thought that it was probably due to a virus infection. The so-called 'rheumatic' stiff neck has nothing to do with rheumatic fever. It is easily distinguished from meningism by the tenderness of muscles in the former, and by the fact that the pain is on lateral or rotary movement and not only on flexion.

Stiffness of the neck, usually but not always without pain, occurs commonly in *rheumatoid arthritis*.

Pain on movement of the neck with stiffness may result from *inflamed cervical lymph nodes* or from a *retropharyngeal abscess*.

Limitation of movement without pain occurs as a feature of *congenital anomalies of the vertebrae*, including fusion of vertebrae. An x-ray photograph will establish the diagnosis. There is also limitation of movement of the neck in the spastic or rigid forms of cerebral palsy. *Myositis ossificans progressiva* commonly begins in the neck muscles; there is a deposition of bone between muscle bundles, gradually spreading through the trunk muscles over a period of years. The bone can readily be felt by the examiner's hand.

If the stiffness of the neck muscles is due to *cerebral palsy*, the other signs of cerebral palsy elsewhere will be obvious.

In the young infant there may be limitation of lateral movement of the neck as a result of a *sternomastoid tumour* (congenital torticollis). The head is pulled and rotated towards the affected side. The tumour can be felt in the sternomastoid muscle.

Neck stiffness and opisthotonos may be a side effect of the phenothiazines.

Reference

DAVIES D.M. (1960) Epidemic cervical myalgia. *Lancet*, **1**, 1275.

Scoliosis

The causes of scoliosis can be classified as follows:

Postural—the scoliosis disappearing when the child bends over
Compensatory—due to unequal length of the legs

Structural—persisting when the child bends over
  Unknown causes
  Muscular dystrophy, late stage
  Poliomyelitis, late effect
  Hemivertebra
  Fragilitas ossium
  Neurofibromatosis involving the spine
  Spina bifida
  Marfan's syndrome
  Congenital heart disease
  Friedreich's ataxia (p. 161)

The clinical diagnosis of most of these conditions is straight-forward, though radiological examination is needed for the diagnosis of hemivertebra and perhaps fragilitas ossium. Marfan's syndrome is diagnosed on the arachnodactyly, tall slender build, subluxation of the lens of the eye and an aortic valve lesion, often with other abnormalities.

Reference

ZORAB P.A. (1969) *Scoliosis*. London, Heinemann.

Facial palsy

The following are the usual causes of facial palsy:

Newborn Babies
  Pressure in utero against the facial nerve
  Injury by forceps
  Nuclear agenesis
  Möbius syndrome. Myotonia dystrophica

Older Children
  Bell's palsy
  Post-ictal
  Mastoiditis

Poliomyelitis
Herpes of the external auditory meatus
Cerebral tumour
Facioscapulohumeral type of muscular dystrophy
Hypertension
Melkersson's syndrome
Cardiofacial syndrome
Guillain-Barré syndrome

The facial palsy of the newborn infant usually clears up in a few weeks. Though facial palsy is usually ascribed to pressure by forceps, it is probable that some cases are of antenatal origin and are caused by pressure in utero against the facial nerve. When the facial palsy does not improve, one suspects the more serious agenesis of the facial nucleus.

The *Möbius syndrome* is also termed congenital facial diplegia. There is striking immobility of the face with hardly any movement, so that the child does not smile and shows little expression when crying. Though the level of intelligence is usually below the average, these children are liable to be considered severely defective when in fact they are only slightly subnormal or even within normal limits. The cause is probably a failure of development of the facial and extraocular muscles. *Myotonia dystrophica* (sometimes called dystrophia myotonica) gives a similar facial appearance. It is characterised by hypotonia, mental retardation, myotonia, progressive muscle wasting, baldness, cataracts and gonadal atrophy. Early weakness in the facial muscles is followed by weakness in the neck, forearm extensors, hand, vasti, quadriceps and ankle dorsiflexors. The mouth tends to hang open and there is a droopy immobile face. The E.M.G. is characteristic.

Facial palsy developing in the older child is usually *Bell's palsy*. It can result from a mastoid infection or from herpes of the external auditory meatus (Ramsay-Hunt Syndrome). The possibility of poliomyelitis should be considered, even though there is no other evidence of paralysis. There may be facial weakness for a few hours after a fit (Todd's paralysis).

Facial palsy of supranuclear type may be due to a *cerebral tumour*, especially a glioma of the pons.

Weakness of the facial muscles may develop in infancy or early childhood in the *facioscapulohumeral type of muscular dystrophy*.

Lloyd, Jewitt, and Still (1966) noted the frequency with which facial paralysis occurs in children with *hypertension*. The facial palsy is of lower motor neurone type. It was found in 20 per cent of 35 severely hypertensive children, possibly as a result of haemorrhage into the facial canal.

Melkersson's syndrome consists of facial palsy, chronic or recurrent oedema of the face and a furrowed tongue.

Cayler described the association of transient facial palsy with *congenital heart disease* and other defects.

Bilateral facial palsy occurs in the *Guillain-Barré syndrome*.

Reference

CAYLER G.G. (1969) Cardiofacial syndrome. *Arch. Dis. Childh.,* **44,** 69.

LLOYD A.V.C., JEWITT D.E. & STILL J.D.L. (1966) Facial paralysis in children with hypertension. *Arch. Dis. Childh.,* **41,** 292.

Hypotonia

The assessment of muscle tone is part of the routine examination of any infant in a welfare clinic or elsewhere. The assessment is made as follows:

(1) Feeling the muscle. The hypotonic muscle, as in a mongol, feels flabby.

(2) Assessing the resistance to passive movement. One tests in particular the elbow, wrist, hip, knee and ankle. In hypertonic children there is increased resistance, and in hypotonic children the resistance is reduced. One has to distinguish voluntary resistance by the child.

(3) Assessing the range of movement. This is increased in the hypotonic child and decreased in the hypertonic child. For instance, in the case of the mongol, who is always hypotonic, having flexed the hip to a right-angle, abduction is so full that both knees will lie flat on the couch—often with the legs extended. Abduction of

the hip is reduced in hypertonia. Dorsiflexion of the ankle is reduced in hypertonia and increased in hypotonia.

(4) One shakes the limb—holding the arm below the elbow and
the leg below the knee. The amount of movement of the hand or
wrist gives a good idea of the muscle tone.

Numerous papers have been written about hypotonic or 'floppy'
infants, and various classifications have been suggested. The classification below is abbreviated and slightly modified from that of
Dubowitz (1968–9).

Hypotonia with weakness

> Neurogenic atrophy: Werdnig Hoffman infantile spinal muscu-
>   lar atrophy
> Congenital myopathies
>   Structural—Central core disease
>   Nemaline myopathy
> Metabolic—Glycogenoses; McCardle's syndrome: Pompe's syn-
>   drome
> Other neuromuscular disorders:
>   Progressive muscular dystrophy
>   Congenital muscular dystrophy
>   Peripheral neuropathies (e.g. Guillain-Barré syndrome)
>   Myasthenia gravis
>   Dystrophia myotonica
>   Injury to the cervical spinal cord
>   Cerebral palsy (hypotonic type)
>   Benign congenital hypotonia

Hypotonia without significant weakness

> Disorders of the central nervous system
>   Mental deficiency
>   Mongolism
>   Lipoidoses
>   Metabolic diseases
> Prader Willi syndrome
> Connective tissue disorders. Marfan's syndrome. Ehlers Danlos
>   syndrome

Metabolic diseases—nutritional, endocrine
   Rickets, coeliac disease, cretinism, gargoylism, hypercalcaemia,
     renal acidosis
Acute illness
Familial dysautonomia (p. 134)

For a full description of these conditions, the reader is referred to the monograph by Dubowitz. Only a few conditions will be described below.

The Werdnig Hoffman syndrome is the most common cause of severe hypotonia with weakness in an infant. The hypotonia is present at birth or develops in the first few weeks. The tendon jerks are usually absent and there may be fasciculation of the tongue. There is marked indrawing of the chest with inspiration. Contractures develop early. Few babies in whom the symptoms develop in the first two months survive beyond their first birthday. The diagnosis is established by muscle biopsy.

There are benign variants of this condition. The Kugelberg-Wehlander syndrome is one of them, occurring mainly in adolescence or later. There is weakness of the proximal muscles of the limb, with fasciculation, loss of reflexes, and characteristic motor nerve conduction and E.M.G. features.

Congenital myopathies may be the cause of infantile hypotonia. The weakness is mainly proximal and it is not progressive. Muscle enzyme studies and the E.M.G. do not help to establish the diagnosis, which depends on the muscle biopsy.

Metabolic causes of weakness with hypotonia include *McCardle's syndrome* of phosphorylase deficiency with cramps on exertion, and *Pompe's glycogenosis*, which closely resembles Werdnig Hoffman's syndrome.

Progressive muscular atrophy (Duchenne's syndrome) is the common form of muscular atrophy, affecting boys. Hypotonia with sucking and swallowing difficulties may be a feature of *myasthenia gravis* of the transitory type in the newborn; it may also be a feature of the rare congenital persistent type.

Injury to the cervical spinal cord, mainly in a breech delivery, may cause considerable hypotonia. The tendon jerks may be absent. The intercostal muscles may be paralysed and the chest is sucked in with each inspiration, while the abdomen bulges out. The child does not cry when the foot is pricked, while the child with Werdnig-Hoffman disease will cry feebly, but may be unable to move the leg because of paralysis.

There is a rare *atonic form of cerebral palsy*, but the diagnosis can usually be made on the basis of exaggerated tendon jerks, a positive stretch reflex, ankle clonus, and an extensor plantar reflex. It is incorrect to apply the term hypotonia to the excessive head lag when a child with cerebral palsy is pulled to the sitting position.

Benign congenital hypotonia is a nonspecific condition. The term denotes hypotonia with weakness which is nonprogressive but which tends to decrease. Affected children may learn to walk by the age of five or six years. Dubowitz considers that with increasing knowledge this term may cease to exist.

Hypotonia without muscle weakness occurs in a wide variety of conditions. It is an invariable feature of *mongolism* and is common in various nonspecific forms of *mental subnormality*. It is found in many cases of *rickets*, some of *scurvy* and in some of the metabolic diseases with *abnormal aminoaciduria*. It occurs with other cerebral conditions, or conditions affecting the brain, such as *hydranencephaly*, the *lipoidoses* and *galactosaemia*. The *Prader-Willi syndrome* is first manifested by hypotonia; obesity develops later (pp. 21, 213).

Of the connective tissue disorders, *Marfan's syndrome* is characterised by arachnodactyly, hyperextensible joints, hypotonia, iridodonesis, congenital heart disease and other abnormalities. The *Ehlers-Danlos syndrome* of cutis hyperelastica may also be associated with hypotonia.

A variety of *metabolic and nutritional diseases* are associated with some degree of hypotonia. *Rickets* is perhaps the most common of these.

It will be seen that the causes of hypotonia are numerous, and that except where the underlying disease such as mongolism is obvious, expert help is needed to establish the diagnosis. The principal diagnostic measures include muscle biopsy with histochemical studies, serum enzyme estimations, electromyography and nerve conduction velocity studies. Without some of these investigations many of the conditions mentioned cannot be diagnosed. It is important to establish the correct diagnosis in order to determine the prognosis and the risk of another child being affected. In certain cases it is important from the point of view of treatment. For instance, corticosteroids may be of value in polymyositis. All cases should therefore be properly investigated. Hypotonia presents a complex difficult problem and expert advice should be sought when faced with it.

References

Dubowitz V. (1969) The floppy infant. *Clinics in Developmental Medicine. No. 31.*
Paine R.S. & Fenichel G.M. (1965) *Clinical Proceedings of the Children's Hospital of the District of Columbia,* **21,** 175.

Weakness of a limb or limbs

The commonest cause of weakness of an arm from birth is Erb's palsy. There is weakness of flexion of the elbow, wrist drop, and the 'chauffeur's tip position' of the hand. The limb is hypotonic— a point of importance, for I have seen it confused with spastic hemiplegia. The hypertonia of the muscles in mild spastic hemiplegia may be so slight that it cannot be detected until the child is older; but in the ipsilateral leg there is likely to be an exaggerated knee jerk and there may be reduced dorsiflexion of the ankle. In cold weather the affected hemiplegic arm and leg are cold as compared with the normal side. In Erb's palsy the biceps jerk is reduced, while in spastic hemiplegia it is increased. After infancy there is no problem, for Erb's palsy almost always disappears within a few days or weeks of birth.

The other obvious cause of weakness of legs in infancy is *meningomyelocele.*

Assuming that the complaint is not merely one of general lassitude, the following conditions in children after infancy would be considered:

Todd's paralysis after an epileptic fit
Hypotonia
Muscular dystrophy
Glycogen storage disease (rare)
Amyotrophic lateral sclerosis (rare)
Peroneal muscular atrophy (rare)
Sulphatide lipoidosis (rare)
Refsum's disease
Diastematomyelia
Effect of an injection
Lipoma of the cauda equina region
Dermatomyositis (p. 38)
Myasthenia gravis (p. 38)
Polyneuritis
Spinal or cerebral tumour or abscess
Poliomyelitis
Guillain-Barré syndrome
Syringomyelia
Hysteria
Drugs

After a major epileptic fit there may be weakness of a limb or of arm and leg, lasting usually for a few hours and occasionally for a few days. (*Todd's paralysis.*)

The first symptom of *muscular dystrophy* is weakness, particularly on climbing stairs in the case of the common pseudohypertrophic variety. The child may begin to walk on his toes. The weakness involves the proximal muscles before the distal ones and the lower limbs before the upper. The various forms of muscular dystrophy and their mode of inheritance were reviewed by Dubowitz (1965). The special investigations commonly required are estimation of the serum creatine phosphokinase, the electromyogram and a muscle biopsy.

If there is generalised weakness of the limbs, one should look for fasciculation in the muscles of the limbs, and for fasciculation and wasting of the tongue muscles. If present, it would indicate an anterior horn cell lesion such as neurogenic muscular atrophy.

Glycogen storage disease Type 2 (Pompe) is manifested by hypotonia from early infancy, large tongue, weakness, mental subnormality and enlargement of the heart. The diagnosis is established by biopsy.

Amyotrophic lateral sclerosis occurs in childhood, but is rare. There is progressive weakness, wasting and fasciculation of the tongue, with loss of reflexes.

Peroneal muscular atrophy is rare: there is weakness of the evertors and dorsiflexors of the feet, followed by loss of reflexes, the development of hammer toes and later involvement of the arms. There may be thickening of the peripheral nerves.

Sulphatide lipoidosis (metachromatic leucodystrophy) is characterised by weakness starting in the first year, hypotonia, mental deterioration, optic atrophy and nystagmus. The motor nerve conduction time is prolonged.

Diastematomyelia is a condition in which the spinal cord is split and tethered by a spicule of bone. It leads to progressive weakness of the legs. It is sometimes revealed by a patch of pigmentation or hair over the spine.

A *lipoma* in the region of the cauda equina is an important cause of progressive weakness of the lower limbs, usually with loss of sphincter control. The lipoma can be seen and palpated in the region of the sacrum or buttock.

Children may develop *polyneuritis*. Tasker and Chutorian (1969) described 17 children between infancy and adolescence with distal muscle weakness and sensory changes. The polyneuritis lasted for varying periods from 16 months to many years. There was decreased nerve conduction time and a raised C.S.F. protein.

Peripheral neuritis may be due to poisons, especially heavy metals, or infections, especially diphtheria.

A *spinal* or *cerebral tumour* or *abscess* should be suspected when there is progressive weakness of a limb or limbs.

Poliomyelitis, the *Guillain-Barré syndrome* and *polyneuritis* would be suspected only in acute cases. In the latter condition the paresis is usually symmetrical. *Syringomyelia* is rare in childhood.

Hysteria is a possible cause of weakness of limbs in an older child.

Various *drugs* may cause weakness of limbs, mostly by causing peripheral neuritis. They include chloroquine, colistin, cyclophosphamide, cycloserine, ethionamide, griseofulvin, pyrazinamide and vincristine. Triamcinolone may cause muscular weakness.

Sudden muscle weakness may be due to poliomyelitis, diphtheria, the Guillain-Barré syndrome, neuromyelitis optica, or epidural abscess. The latter is commonly characterised by fever, back pain, stiff neck, and flaccid paralysis of the legs with loss of reflexes.

Weakness due to spasticity or hypertonia is nearly always a manifestation of *cerebral palsy*. The differential diagnosis depends on the distribution of the spasticity. If a child with spastic quadriplegia has been spastic from birth, the cause would almost certainly be cerebral palsy—but if he was normal at first and then became spastic, other causes must be considered. If the disease was of acute onset, it could be due to encephalitis (such as a postinfectious encephalomyelitis), or to an intracranial vascular accident, such as thrombosis due to dehydration. If the spasticity is of gradual onset, it may be due to one of the numerous degenerative diseases of the nervous system, such as Schilder's disease—which is manifested by the gradual development of blindness, deafness and spasticity beginning in early childhood. There are so many degenerative diseases of the nervous system that it would be impossible to review them all here. The reader should refer to any of the textbooks of paediatric neurology, such as that of Ford (1966). Other causes of progressive spasticity involving all four limbs include craniovertebral abnormalities, such as basilar impression and the Klippel-Feil syndrome of fused cervical vertebrae with other anomalies. Neuromyelitis optica and its near relative disseminated sclerosis are other causes of spasticity of rapid onset. It should be noted that the spasticity of cerebral palsy may increase as the child grows older, and the development of deformities, such as dislocation of the hip and joint fixation due to muscle contracture may give a false impression that the child has a progressive neurological disorder.

When the spasticity of cerebral palsy is almost entirely confined to the lower limbs, it is easy to diagnose spastic paraplegia, while more careful examination of the upper limbs when the child is building a tower of bricks or performing a timed bead-threading test, will show that there is minimal involvement of the upper limbs, so that the true diagnosis is cerebral diplegia. True spastic paraplegia is rare, and should alert one to the possibility that the lesion is spinal and not cerebral. The spinal lesion may be a tumour, cyst or other anomaly, and it should be looked for, because it may be treatable. Diastematomyelia (p. 214) is one of the possible causes of progressive weakness of the lower limbs. As there may be signs of pyramidal tract involvement, this should be looked for. There may or may not be a helpful patch of hair or pigmentation over the affected area.

References

DUBOWITZ V. (1965) Muscular dystrophy and related disorders. *Postgrad. med. J.*, **41**, 332.

DUBOWITZ V., LORBER J. & ZACHARY R.B. (1965) Lipoma of the cauda equina. *Arch. Dis. Childh.*, **40**, 207.

TASKER W. & CHUTORIAN A.M. (1969) Chronic polyneuritis of childhood. *J. Pediat.*, **74**, 667.

Excessive muscle tone

The main conditions which should be considered are the following:

Normal variations in early infancy
Cerebral palsy

Many infants in the first days and weeks have greater than usual muscle tone with exaggerated tendon jerks and often with ankle clonus. Unless there are other abnormal signs, such as smallness of the head circumference in relation to the baby's weight or delayed motor development, one pays little attention to it. The signs usually disappear as the child grows older.

The commonest cause of persistently excessive muscle tone is *cerebral palsy*. The commonest type to be associated with excessive tone is the spastic variety. The tendon jerks are exaggerated, there may be ankle clonus and the plantar responses are extensor. There is excessive muscle tone in many children with the athetoid form, and in all with the so-called rigid form, which is always associated with mental deficiency of severe degree.

Excessive muscle tone, restricting the range of movement in a joint, may be confused with *deformities of joints*, such as arthrogryposis or other congenital abnormalities. Reduced range of movement in a joint such as the hip could be ascribed to increased muscle tone, when it is due to contracture of the muscles, as a result of the child (usually severely mentally defective or hypotonic) always lying in one position.

The *development of excessive muscle tone in a previously normal child* suggests the following possibilities:

Encephalitis or meningitis if acute, and other infections of the central nervous system
Demyelinating or degenerative disease of the nervous system
Cerebral or spinal abscess or tumour
Drugs

The number of conditions involved is so considerable, covering a large section of the whole of paediatric neurology, that it would not be profitable to discuss these here. An affected child should be investigated by a paediatrician.

Toe walking

Some *normal toddlers* walk on their toes by habit. There are no signs of spasticity or other disease.

A *prematurely born baby* on reaching what would have been term is liable to bear his weight on his toes rather than on the sole of his foot.

By far the commonest cause of toe walking is *cerebral palsy of the spastic type*. If the toe walking is unilateral, there will be the usual signs of spastic hemiplegia—the characteristic gait, shortening of the affected leg and arm, some wasting of the affected limbs, limited dorsiflexion of the affected ankle, relative coldness of the affected limbs as compared with the normal ones, limited abduction of the hip, exaggerated knee jerk and plantar extensor response on the affected side, and possibly ankle clonus. If both lower limbs are involved, there will almost certainly be signs of at least slight involvement of the arms, if the child is old enough to perform fine repetitive movements.

An unusual cause is *congenital shortening of the Tendo Achillis*. The absence of other signs of cerebral palsy and especially of an exaggerated knee jerk, limited abduction of the hip or of an extensor plantar response, should make a mistaken diagnosis unnecessary.

An early sign of *dystonia musculorum deformans* is often toe-walking ('The ballet-dancer's foot'). (See p. 183.)

Other causes of toe-walking are *infantile autism, muscular dystrophy, peroneal muscular atrophy* (p. 214) and a *spinal cord tumour*.

Limp and limb pains

When a previously well child begins to limp, one examines the shoe for a protruding nail, crinkling of the sole or excessive tightness; one then examines the child's lower limbs for a sore place or bone tenderness (due to fracture), not forgetting to look for enlarged tender inguinal lymph nodes. One then examines the ankle and knee joints for pain on movement and heat on palpation, and the hip joint in order to determine whether the range of movement, particularly in abduction and rotation, is full and painless. One remembers the frequency with which pain in the knee is pain referred from a diseased hip.

Finally one examines the spine for the range of movement, and the abdomen, in case the limp is related to psoas spasm due to intra-abdominal inflammation.

The following are the more important bone and joint conditions affecting children and liable to present as a limp or limb pain:

Trauma, soft tissue injury, fracture, sprains and twists
Traumatic periostitis
Caffey's disease in the newborn
Transient synovitis of the hip

Osteochondritis
  Perthes' disease of the hip
  Kohler's disease of the tarsal navicular
  Osgood Schlatter's disease of the tibial tuberosity
  Freiburg's disease of the metatarsal head
  Scheuermann's disease of the spine
Discitis
Spondylitis
Slipped femoral epiphysis
Arthritis, joint effusions, and osteitis
Congenital dislocation of the hip
Spastic hemiplegia
Congenital asymmetry
Inequality of length of limb
Leukaemia and Hodgkin's disease
Growing pains (p. 226)
Poliomyelitis
Soft tissue infection (e.g. following intramuscular injection)
Bone tumour or cyst
Scurvy
Sickle cell anaemia
Attention-seeking devices
Hypervitaminosis A
Collagen disease
Muscle pain from injury; myositis, trichinosis
Muscle cramps—McCardle's syndrome
                 Effect of drugs
                 Dehydration
Spine—osteitis, spondilolisthesis

A limp at the age of one to two years is more likely to be due to injury, congenital subluxation of the hip or spastic hemiplegia. At the age of two to five years, trauma, spastic hemiplegia or transient synovitis of hip; from the age of five to ten years, trauma, transient synovitis of hip, Perthes' or Kohler's disease; and from ten to 15 years a slipped upper femoral epiphysis, Osgood-Schlatter's disease or hysteria.

When an older child complains of vague limb and back pains,

and no abnormal physical signs can be found, one should remember the possibility that the pain may result from a variety of *vigorous childhood pursuits*, such as hula-hoop, violent games, dances of the Twist variety and physical training.

Traumatic periostitis may result from a twist or sprain of a limb. Recovery is usually complete within seven to ten days. An x-ray may show a periosteal reaction about a week after the injury.

Caffey's disease of the newborn presents as tender swellings over the bones, particularly the jaws and lower limbs. The cause is unknown, but there may be a genetic factor. Recovery is complete. The diagnosis is confirmed by the x-ray, which shows periosteal elevation.

Transient synovitis of the hip is common, but its exact pathological nature is not well understood. Stock (1959) and Jacobs (1971) have reviewed the condition, describing 109 cases. The age of onset ranges from 18 months to seven years, with a peak incidence of six years. It is more common in boys. In two-thirds it follows an upper respiratory tract infection, and in one-sixth it follows injury. It is more common in obese children. The symptom is a limp or pain in the hip of acute onset, with limitation of movement. The average duration of symptoms is 13 days, and recovery is complete within two months. Weight-bearing during the acute stage prolongs the symptoms. Special investigations do not help, except an x-ray to exclude more serious conditions. The white cell count is normal. The erythrocyte sedimentation rate is normal or only slightly raised. The x-ray of the hip does not show any abnormality.

The most common form of *osteochondritis* in the lower limbs is Perthes' disease of the hip. The age of onset is most commonly two to ten years. It presents with limitation of hip movement and a limp, with very little pain or no pain at all. It is bilateral in 10 per cent. On examination there is limitation of abduction in particular, and of external rotation and extension of the hip. The diagnosis is confirmed by x-ray of the hip. There may be wasting of the glutei and flat buttocks. The diagnosis of the other forms of osteochondritis listed depends on the x-ray.

For discitis and spondylitis see p. 230.

Slipped femoral epiphysis occurs especially between the age of ten and 15 years. It is more common in boys, especially when tall and fat. It is bilateral in 20 per cent. The symptom is a limp with little pain. On examination there is limited abduction of the hip.

Congenital dislocation of the hip should have been diagnosed long before the child walked. If the diagnosis has been missed, the child usually presents with a limp due partly to the apparent shortening of the leg.

The following conditions increase the risk that a child will have dislocation of the hip:

Family history
Geographical factors (it is especially common in Northern Italy)
Breech delivery
Severe spasticity
Severe hypotonia, e.g. meningomyelocele, amyotonia
Bilateral talipes, especially female
Arthrogryposis

The clinical diagnosis can be readily made by the finding of limited abduction of the hip and shortening of the leg with a characteristic waddling gait. The diagnosis is confirmed by x-ray of the hip.

Inequality in the length of a limb is due to spastic hemiplegia, old poliomyelitis, or congenital asymmetry. A limb may be abnormally large as a result of an *angiomatous malformation*.

The condition termed *congenital asymmetry, hemihypertrophy,* or *hemiatrophy* is a complex one, associated with mental deficiency in about a third, and often with other abnormalities such as dysmaturity, short stature, retarded bone age, short incurved little finger, syndactyly, and a turning down at the angle of the mouth. In others it is associated with abnormalities of the retina, or with neurofibromatosis and Wilms's tumour. In some cases it has been found that there is an increased gonadotrophin excretion in the urine, with early puberty. The whole of one side of the body, including the bones, is larger than the other.

Leukaemia and *Hodgkin's disease* are important causes of bone pain. They should certainly be considered when a child complains of pain in bone.

Poliomyelitis may cause severe limb pain in the preparalytic stage, due to spasm in the muscles about to be paralysed. There is likely to be reduction or loss of the relevant tendon jerks.

Scurvy causes acute pain in the limb of the young infant or child, due to subperiosteal haemorrhage. It now occurs in Britain mainly in defective children in whom it has been difficult to maintain nutrition. There is usually sponginess of the gums.

Sickle cell anaemia may be responsible for severe pain in a limb, sometimes associated with osteitis.

Myalgia may result from trichinosis, due to eating uncooked meat. Symptoms include fever and orbital oedema. There is usually eosinophilia. The diagnosis is confirmed by an intradermal test and biopsy of the deltoid muscle.

McCardle's syndrome consists of muscle fatigue and cramps on exertion. It is due to deficiency of muscle phosphorylase.

Various *drugs* may cause limb pains. Cramp may be caused by lincomycin, nalidixic acid, sulphasalazine and the thiazide diuretics.

Limb pains may be caused by rifampicin. Barbiturates and penicillin may cause a serum sickness type of reaction with effusion into joints. Rubella immunisation may cause arthritis. Various drugs may cause disseminated lupus erythromatosus (p. 33) and sulphonamides may cause polyarteritis—both conditions which may cause limb discomfort.

Cramps may also be due to heat stroke, or to sodium loss resulting from *dehydration*.

Attention seeking device. I have known children in hospital develop a limp because they did not want to go home. A limp may be feigned to avoid going to school.

Hypervitaminosis A is due to excessive doses of vitamin A. It causes angular stomatitis, sore tongue, hepatomegaly and bone pains due to periostitis.

References

Adverse Drug Reaction Bulletin (1971). *Drug induced aches and pains*. No. 30, p. 88.

BARLOW T.H. (1962) Early diagnosis and treatment of congenital dislocation of the hip. *J. Bone and Joint Surgery*, 44 B, 292.

JACOBS B.W. (1971) Synovitis of the hip in children and its significance. *Pediatrics*, 47, 558.

RINGROSE R.E., JABBOUR J.T. & KEELE D.K. (1965) Hemihypertrophy. *Pediat.*, 36, 434.
STOCK A. (1959) Transient synovitis of the hip joint in children. *Pediat.*, 24, 1042.

Arthritis and joint pains

The common causes of arthritis or pain in the joints are as follows:

Trauma and joint strain
Henoch-Schönlein purpura
Sickle cell anaemia
Rheumatic fever
Rheumatoid arthritis
Steroid pseudorheumatism
Haemophilia and Christmas disease

Other causes include the following:

Osteitis and pyogenic arthritis
Osteochondritis
Spondylitis, discitis
Meningococcal septicaemia
Tuberculosis
Syphilis
Sarcoid
Serum sickness
Rubella or rubella immunisation
Dysentery, salmonella infections, typhoid fever
Ulcerative colitis and Crohn's disease
Glandular fever
Brucellosis
Psoriasis
Disseminated lupus
Gout
Drugs

Pain in the joints (unless purely psychogenic) may be due to *joint* strain caused by dances of the 'Twist' variety, or other violent pursuits of youth, apart from actual fractures near the joint.

Henoch-Schönlein purpura (*allergic purpura*) is commonly accompanied by effusion into joints (p. 54).

Sickle cell anaemia may present as acute arthritis or dactylitis.

Rheumatic fever is now becoming much less common in Britain. Its main features are arthritis, lassitude, fever and often carditis, following (in about a third of all cases) a known previous throat infection. In the remaining two thirds the streptococcal infection may be proved by estimation of the anti-streptolysin O titre and culture of haemolytic streptococci from the throat swab. The arthritis is typically a 'flitting polyarthritis', involving mainly (and almost entirely) the knee, ankle, wrist and elbow, only occasionally the hip, and rarely other joints. Hip involvement in rheumatic fever is unusual. The arthritis starts in one joint and clears after two or three days, moving to other joints in rotation, but the arthritis may involve one joint only or at least treatment is given so promptly that other joints are not involved. Occasionally there may be a mere complaint of pain in joints without any detectable arthritis. In my experience all children with arthritis due to rheumatic fever are unwell. If a child complains of pains in the joints and yet feels well and full of energy, rheumatic fever can be almost excluded. Fever may be short-lasting and subside before the child is referred to the doctor. The ESR is invariably high (unless there is heart failure due to carditis, in which case the ESR is normal in about a quarter of all cases). If the ESR was not very high (e.g. if it were merely 15 to 20 mm in an hour, micro Westergren method), I would exclude the diagnosis of rheumatic fever as a cause of the arthritis. Other useful investigations are the antistreptolysin O titre (which should be over 200 units) and the presence of C reactive protein (CRP). Both these tests are positive in almost a hundred per cent of cases in the acute stage.

There is almost always a raised sleeping pulse rate in the early stage (e.g. over 100 per minute), but there is often a sinus bradycardia (e.g. pulse rate of 60 per minute) in the early convalescent stage. If the pulse rate is fast, the sleeping pulse rate alone is of value, because tachycardia due to emotional factors must be excluded. The murmur of an obvious carditis may clinch the diagnosis; but in the early stage of such a murmur it is essential to distinguish a functional murmur. Almost one in two of all children have an innocent murmur. In many, the diagnosis is obvious: in others considerable clinical experience is needed to satisfy oneself that the murmur is not organic in origin. A child with fever, hyperthyroidism, severe anaemia or marked tachycardia may have an innocent murmur. It is not easy to describe in words the difference between a functional and an organic murmur. The functional murmur is either soft or musical and high pitched. It is commonly of short duration, tends to be late in systole, to be louder when the child lies down than when he is upright, and is often increased by exertion. Some describe the murmur as being on occasion 'vibratory' or 'twanging' in character. Functional murmurs are not confined to any one part of the heart. They may be mainly apical, along the sternal border or at the base.

Duckett Jones in the United States devised criteria for the establishment of the diagnosis of rheumatic fever. These were subsequently modified by the American Heart Association and the Medical Research Council, as follows:

Major criteria
(1) Carditis, revealed by:
    (a) Development of an organic apical systolic murmur or an aortic diastolic murmur under observation
    (b) Change in heart size of more than 15 per cent on a standard x-ray film
    (c) Pericarditis, shown by rub or effusion
    (d) Congestive failure under the age of 25 years, without other cause
(2) Polyarthritis
(3) Chorea
(4) Rheumatic nodules
(5) Erythema marginatum

Minor criteria
1) Fever—99.3° or more (by mouth)
2) Raised ESR

(3) Evidence of haemolytic streptococcal infection, as shown by the history, ASO titre or throat swab.
(4) Increased PR interval in the ECG
(5) Past history of rheumatic fever

The diagnosis of rheumatic fever was to be based on the presence of two major criteria, or one major and two minor criteria. In practice this method of diganosis has worked well, but an occasional child with rheumatic fever does not satisfy the criteria, and an occasional child with some other condition does satisfy them.

I have seen many children who were thought to have rheumatic fever when in fact they had *febrile aches and pains in the limbs*. These occur in any infection associated with fever and are non-articular.

Many children are thought to have rheumatic fever when they have *'growing-pains'*—a misnomer, because the pains occur predominantly before the period of maximum growth. Apley found that one in every twenty-five Bristol school children had such pains. They are non-articular pains, involving mainly the thigh and calf muscles, and occur mainly at night in bed. Their cause is unknown. The ESR is normal, an important fact which entirely eliminates rheumatic fever as a cause. Øster and Nielsen (1972) in a study of 2,178 school children aged 6 to 19 years, found that the peak age of growing pains was 11, and at that age approximately 20 per cent of the boys and 30 per cent of the girls complained of them. The overall incidence in boys was 12·5 per cent and in girls 18·4 per cent. Twenty-eight per cent of those with growing pains also had headaches and 22 per cent had abdominal pains, either simultaneously or at different times. The children were otherwise normal.

I have seen children with pain from other causes, such as *incipient poliomyelitis*, thought to have rheumatic fever.

It is important that the correct diagnosis should be made in order that the appropriate treatment, corticosteroids and salicylates, can be given in hospital.

Rheumatoid arthritis

The peak age of onset of rheumatoid arthritis is two to four years, though it may begin long before two—even in the first year. It is more common in girls than in boys. The presenting symptom is usually pain in a joint. A troublesome presenting symptom or sign, which may last for some months before a joint becomes involved, is unexplained fever. This occurs in some ten per cent of all cases. A single joint may be involved or several joints may be painful at one time. When a single joint is involved, it is most likely to be a knee or ankle. The joint becomes enlarged, movement is painful and becomes restricted, and the joint is hot on palpation. There are signs of effusion into the joint. About half of all cases present with involvement of a single joint, and over a period of months no other joint may be involved. Involvement of the small joints of the fingers (especially the proximal interphalangeal joints) is a common and characteristic feature of other cases. There is commonly wasting of the muscles surrounding an affected joint. Muscle weakness is a common complaint. In about a quarter of all cases there is a characteristic salmon pink maculopapular slightly raised rash, consisting of lesions one to two cms in diameter, sometimes oval in shape with a pale centre. The lesions appear mainly in the latter part of the day, especially on the extremities. The incidence of splenic and lymph node enlargement in rheumatoid arthritis is often exaggerated. It occurs in not more than one in ten of all affected children.

It may be difficult to distinguish rheumatoid arthritis from rheumatic fever. Rheumatic nodules may occur in both. The following are the main differentiating points in doubtful cases:

(1) Stiffness in the mornings strongly favours the diagnosis of rheumatoid arthritis.

(2) Duration of joint involvement. Arthritis in one joint does not last more than a few days in rheumatic fever, even if no treatment is given.

(3) Involvement of the neck and proximal interphalangeal joints suggests rheumatoid arthritis.

(4) A normal ESR, a negative ASO titre, or the absence of CRP, excludes the diagnosis of rheumatic fever. The ESR is normal in 30 to 40 per cent of children with active rheumatoid arthritis. A high ESR (over 40 mm in an hour, using the micro-Westergren method) is unusual in rheumatoid arthritis; an ESR between 10 and 20 mm

would exclude the diagnosis of rheumatic fever with arthritis unless there were heart failure. The ASO titre is negative in 80 per cent of children with rheumatoid arthritis, and CRP is absent in 70 per cent. These tests are positive in 99 per cent of children with rheumatic fever and arthritis.

(5) Iridocyclitis. This occurs in about 15 per cent of children with rheumatoid arthritis.

(6) If the child is under five, he would almost certainly be ill if he had rheumatic fever and would have obvious carditis. I would almost exclude rheumatic fever if a four-year-old had arthritis without carditis. Under the age of three, rheumatic fever is exceedingly rare. Unfortunately tests for the rheumatoid factor do not often help in children. The tests are rarely positive in the absence of rheumatic nodules. Where it is important to establish the diagnosis in a child with prolonged joint involvement, a biopsy of the synovial membrane is useful.

When corticosteroids are discontinued after prolonged administration (e.g. for asthma, rheumatoid arthritis), there may be joint pains, stiffness, paraesthesiae and malaise (Hargreave *et al.*, 1969).

Haemophilia and Christmas disease may be associated with haemorrhage in the joints.

Pyogenic arthritis or osteitis near a joint can readily be confused with rheumatic fever. The diagnosis is made more difficult when two or three joints are involved in osteitis. When there is any doubt at all (as there often is), a blood culture should be taken before any penicillin is given.

For spondylitis and discitis see p. 230.

Meningococcal septicaemia is commonly associated with joint involvement.

Tuberculosis of a joint is diagnosed by a tuberculin reaction and x-ray changes. A negative reaction eliminates tuberculosis except when there is miliary spread, or temporary anergy in an acute illness such as measles, or in the very early pre-allergic phase.

Eleven cases of *sarcoid arthritis* were described by North *et al.* (1970). They were characterised by large painless boggy synovial and tendon sheath effusions involving the wrists, ankles, knees and elbows, little limitation of movement, chronic course with minimal constitutional symptoms, in association with uveitis but without hilar lymphadenopathy, hypergammaglobulinaemia (except in one case) and with no abnormality in laboratory findings apart from a raised E.S.R. There was a slow successive involvement of joints over a two to three year period. The onset in all eleven was before the age of four years. The writers noted that the extent of the swelling would be unusual in rheumatoid arthritis, as would the absence of slight degree of pain, stiffness or limitation of movement.

Serum sickness is commonly associated with joint effusion. It follows seven to ten days after the injection of diphtheria or tetanus antitoxin, and is associated with fever, rash and lymphadenopathy. A similar picture may result from allergy to penicillin or other drug.

Arthritis may result from *dysentery, salmonella infections, typhoid fever, rubella, brucellosis, ulcerative colitis, Crohn's disease* or *psoriasis.* Mild arthralgia may accompany almost any type of *drug induced general rash.* Barbiturates, methimazole and penicillin may cause a joint effusion. It may follow rubella immunisation.

Disseminated lupus erythematosus may closely resemble rheumatoid arthritis. The possibility of a child having *juvenile gout,* particularly if there is a family history of that complaint, should be remembered. It may be primary or secondary to leukaemia or haemolytic anaemia.

References

Adverse Drug Reaction Bulletin (1971). Drug induced aches and pains. No. 30, p. 88.

British Medical Journal (1972) Juvenile gout. Leading article. **1,** 129.

CASTLE R.F. (1961) Clinical recognition of innocent cardiac murmurs in children. *J. Am. Med. Ass.,* **177,** 1.

CONNELLY J.P. (1965) Arthritis in Childhood. *Clin. Pediatrics,* **4,** 215.

HARGREAVE F.E., MCCARTHY D.S. & PEPYS J. (1969) Steroid pseudorheumatism in asthma. *Brit. med. J.,* **1,** 443.

JONES T.D. (1944) The diagnosis of rheumatic fever. *J. Am. Med. Ass.,* **126,** 481.

LAAKSONEN A. (1966) A prognostic study of juvenile rheumatoid arthritis. Analysis of 544 cases. *Acta Paediat Scandinavica, Suppl.,* 166.

LEVINE S.A. & HARVEY W.P. (1950) *Clinical ausculation of the heart.* Philadelphia, Saunders.

NORTH A.F., FINK C.W., GIBSON W.M., LEVINSON J.E., SCHUCTER S.L., HOWARD W.K., JOHNSON N.H. & HARRIS C. (1970) Sarcoid arthritis in children. *Am. J. Med.,* **48,** 449.

Øster J. & Nielsen A. (1972) Growing Pains. *Acta. Paediat. Scandinav.*, **61**, 329.
Wasz-Hockert O., Stenman U. & Kostia J. (1965) Monoarthritis in children. *Ann. Paediat Fenniae*, **11**, 119.

Back pain

The commonest cause of back pain in children is ligamentous strain or intervertebral disc lesions in the lumbosacral spine or neck. They are usually due to athletic and gymnastic exercises to which the child is not accustomed or perhaps suited. According to my colleague J. Sharrard F.R.C.S., who has helped me with this section, intervertebral disc lesions are not uncommon in children, but are rarely recognised. The so-called fibrositis is probably non-existent; the symptoms are probably due to ligamentous strain or pain referred from the disc region.

Back pain and related symptoms have been ascribed to *discitis*. Menelaus (1964) described 35 cases seen at the Royal Children's Hospital, Melbourne. The youngest was ten months old. Symptoms included abdominal pain, vomiting, malaise, back pain, stiff neck, vague pain in the buttocks, knee or thigh, or a limp. On examination there was lordosis, stiffness of the back and sometimes fever and local tenderness. The E.S.R. was sometimes raised. The x-ray showed narrowing of the disc space.

Ankylosing spondylitis may begin in childhood, and is more common in boys. The initial symptoms are characteristically fleeting and recurrent, and consist of pain, stiffness and lack of mobility in the back, with vague pains in the buttocks, thighs and hips. There may be transient pain in the large joints. It must be distinguished from *rheumatoid arthritis* (p. 226), in which low back pain is unusual, cervical involvement is more common, and the arthritis is more persistent; and from *Scheuermann's* disease of the spine, mainly thoracic, a cause of adolescent kyphosis and back pain. Other conditions which could cause confusion are discitis and Perthes' disease of the hip.

Spondylolisthesis, spinal tumours and developmental disorders of the spine may also cause back pain.

References

MENELAUS M.B. (1964) Discitis. *J. Bone and Joint Surgery*, **46B**, 16.
SCHALLER J., BITNUM S. & WEDGWOOD R.J. (1969) Ankylosing spondylitis with childhood onset. *J. Pediat.*, **74**, 505.

Local muscle wasting

The usual causes of local muscle wasting are the following:
Spastic hemiplegia
Injections
Nerve injuries, by section or pressure
Diseases of the central nervous system
Poliomyelitis, spina bifida, diastematomyelia, tumour, syringomyelia
Polyneuritis, including that due to drugs
Muscular dystrophy
Peroneal muscular atrophy

It has to be distinguished from the following conditions:
Lipodystrophy
Congenital absence of muscle, such as the pectoralis major
Congenital asymmetry (hemihypertrophy, hemiatrophy)

The limbs involved in *spastic hemiplegia* are wasted, but not markedly so, and not nearly as much as a limb affected by poliomyelitis.

Local muscle wasting may result from *injections*, either by damage to a nerve or by direct effect on a muscle. Those involved are usually the radial or sciatic nerves. Because of the risk of damage to nerves, no intramuscular injection should ever be made into the arm. The outer aspect of the thigh is a safer place for an injection than the buttocks.

Local wasting may result from a variey of *neurological conditions*, such as *poliomyelitis, spina bifida, diastematomyelia, congenital dermal sinus, sacrococcygeal lipoma, spinal tumour* or *syringomyelia*.

Polyneuritis may occur without known cause. It may follow acute infectious diseases, especially diphtheria, or certain drugs, in particular chloramphenicol, isoniazid, nalidixic acid or nitrofurantoin. It may follow lead poisoning, serum sickness, tetanus toxoid or malnutrition. It may follow an injection of tetanus toxoid.

There may be local wasting in *muscular dystrophy* (e.g. scapulohumeral type).

Peroneal muscular atrophy is a hereditary disease associated with wasting in the distal muscles, with weakness and loss of reflexes. Wasting and weakness commonly begin in the feet, progressing slowly to the peroneal and later to the calf muscles. Wasting rarely occurs above the knee. There may be fasciculation in the muscle.

Local muscle wasting must be distinguished from *lipodystrophy, congenital absence of muscle* and *congenital asymmetry*. Lipodystrophy commonly affects the face in the first place, but may be confined to the lower limbs. As the term implies, there is a loss of fat but not of muscle.

Congenital absence of muscle, such as that of the pectoralis major (p. 239) could be confused with muscle wasting. Congenital asymmetry (hemihypertrophy, hemiatrophy) is mentioned on p. 221.

Asymmetry of the head

By far the commonest causes of asymmetry of the head and face (other than facial palsy) are posture and congenital asymmetry. Craniostenosis and a partial Treacher-Collins syndrome are rare causes. It is extremely common to find that a young baby's head is flat on one side, because he has consistently lain on that side, while it bulges out at the other side. The skull becomes more symmetrical as he grows older, and no treatment is necessary.

Many babies are born with some degree of cranial asymmetry, and it is of no importance.

Extreme asymmetry may be due to craniostenosis—premature closure of the cranial sutures. As this can be treated by the surgeon, a child suspected of having craniostenosis should be referred to an expert for advice.

On rare occasions severe asymmetry may be due to a partial Treacher-Collins syndrome or other rare anomaly of the first arch.

A small head

The size of the head is closely related to the size of the cranial contents. If the brain does not grow normally, the head is likely to be unusually small. Hence the measurement of the head circumference is an important part of the developmental assessment of an infant, in that it may add confirmatory evidence of defective mental development or of early hydrocephalus. The measurement of the head circumference should be just as much part of the routine examination of any baby in a baby clinic, doctor's surgery or hospital, as is the examination of the hips for congenital subluxation, of the urine for phenylpyruvic acid, of the back for a congenital dermal sinus, and—after three or four months—a rough test of hearing.

It is easy to make an erroneous diagnosis of microcephaly and therefore of mental deficiency when in fact the child is normal. It is necessary to be aware of the other causes of smallness of the head circumference.

When a child has an unusually small head, one should consider the following conditions:

Normal variation
Small baby
Familial feature
Microcephaly
Craniostenosis

A small baby is likely to have a smaller head than a big baby, and a big baby is likely to have a bigger head than a small baby. Hence the maximum head circumference must be related to the size of the baby. This can be done by plotting the head circumference and the weight on the relevant centile charts. The two normally coincide, though a small or large head may be a familial feature which affects the position on the chart. Hence when the head is unusual, one must see both parents.

The fact that the head circumference corresponds exactly with the fiftieth centile by no means suggest that the head is normal. The

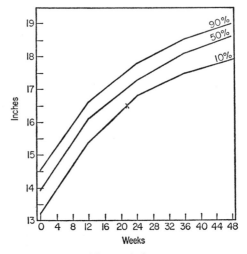

(a) Head chart
Small head corresponding to weight

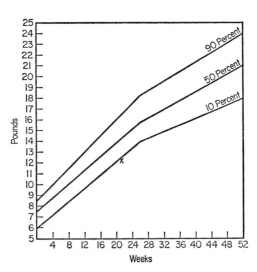

(b) Weight chart
Head size corresponds to weight

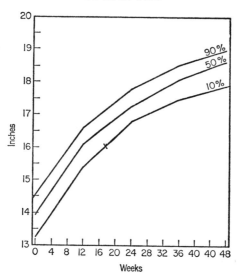

(c) Head chart

Microcephaly. Head small in relation to weight

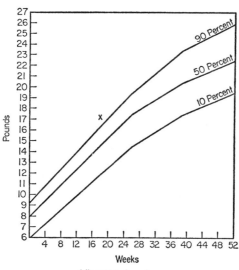

(d) Weight chart

Microcephaly. Same child

child might have microcephaly if he is a particularly big baby, or hydrocephalus if he is a particularly small baby.

When there is true microcephaly, the head is not only unusually small, but it is badly shaped, tapering off towards the vertex.

Craniostenosis or premature closure of the cranial sutures is a rare cause of undue smallness of the head. The fused sutures may be palpated by the experienced finger, but the diagnosis is established by x-ray. The anterior fontanelle would be closed.

A large head

When a baby has an unusually large head, the following conditions should be considered:

Normal variation
Large baby
Familial feature
Hydrocephalus
Megalencephaly
Hydranencephaly
Subdural effusion
Cerebral tumour or cyst
Cerebral gigantism (rare) and other rare conditions

The first two of these have already been discussed.

An unusually large head may indicate hydrocephalus. The diagnosis would be confirmed by the finding of a bulging fontanelle, widely separated sutures, serial measurements plotted on a head chart which indicate that the head circumference is increasing abnormally fast, and air studies. Rare causes are cerebral gigantism (early excessive growth in height, acromegalic features, prominent forehead, large hands and feet and mental retardation): achondroplasia, in which the head is usually somewhat large: sulphatide lipoidosis (p. 214), or gangliosidosis. It is important that such a child should be sent promptly to a specialist in order that the hydrocephalus can be treated. This prevents the development of mental deficiency and blindness from optic atrophy.

It is important to note that two errors are commonly made in the diagnosis of hydrocephalus. Firstly, a *premature baby* has a relatively large head. Secondly, an older infant (*e.g.* nine to twelve months of age), with the *failure to thrive syndrome*, has a relatively large head.

Megalencephaly is a rare condition in which the child has an unusually large brain of poor quality without hydrocephalus. The diagnosis can only be made by air encephalography.

Hydranencephaly is a rare condition in which the head is full of cerebrospinal fluid with little brain tissue. The diagnosis is established by transillumination in a darkened room and by air studies.

References

ILLINGWORTH R.S. & LUTZ W. (1965) The measurement of the infant's head circumference and its significance. *Arch. Dis. Childh.*, **40**, 672.

ILLINGWORTH R.S. (1972) *The development of the infant and young child, normal and abnormal*, Edinburgh, Churchill Livingstone.

ILLINGWORTH R.S. & EID E. (1971) Head circumference in relation to weight, chest circumference, supine length and crown rump length in the first six months of life, *Acta Paediat. Scand.*, **60**, 333.

Torticollis

The main causes of torticollis are as follows:

Congenital (sternomastoid tumour)
Habit
Cervical adenitis
Ocular torticollis
Myositis
Abnormalities of the cervical spine
Sprengel's deformity (elevation of scapula)
Klippel-Feil syndrome
Vertebral osteitis
Weakness of neck muscles (e.g. poliomyelitis)
Posterior fossa tumour

Hysteria
Spasmodic torticollis (p. 183)
Spasmus nutans (p. 183)
Trauma
Drugs

A baby sometimes holds the head on one side for no apparent reason, and without a sternomastoid tumour.

Congenital torticollis, due to a sternomastoid tumour, is due either to pressure in utero against the sternomastoid muscle or to damage of the muscle during delivery. The hard tumour in the muscle is felt a few days after birth, and torticollis with rotation of the neck develops shortly after.

In an older child, a painful *cervical adenitis*, especially if there is suppuration, may cause torticollis.

Ocular torticollis is a posture adopted by the child to maintain binocular vision and avoid a squint when there is paresis of ocular muscles. The head is tilted and rotated.

The so-called *'rheumatic stiff neck'* may be due to a virus infection; there is tenderness on pressure on the neck muscles. *Myositis ossificans* may begin as a stiff neck with *torticollis*.

It is important to examine the neck in order to determine whether there is a congenital abnormality of the cervical vertebrae, such as that in the *Klippel-Feil syndrome*. The diagnosis will be established by the shortness of the neck and the x-ray. Limited rotation, flexion or extension suggests the need of an x-ray to establish the diagnosis. The fixed high scapula of *Sprengel's deformity* can be seen if looked for.

Vertebral osteitis would probably be associated with pain and tenderness over the bone. An x-ray should be taken when in doubt.

A *posterior fossa tumour* may cause torticollis.

The possibility of *hysteria* as a cause should be considered only when there is no evidence of organic disease and when there is positive evidence of hysteria.

Snyder (1969) described 12 cases of *paroxysmal torticollis* in infants aged two to eight months. They experienced two to three attacks a month of torticollis, crying, pallor and vomiting on rotation of the head; the attacks lasted 10 minutes to 14 days. There was spon-

taneous recovery by the age of five. It was suggested that the cause
was a labyrinthitis or vestibular neuronitis.

Torticollis may be due to *spinal injury*—a rotatory subluxation
between the axis and the atlas, or subluxation of C2 or C3.

The *phenothiazines* may cause torticollis and opisthotonos.

Reference

SNYDER C.H. (1969) Paroxysmal torticollis in infancy. *Am. J. Dis. Child.*, **117**, 458.

Asymmetry of the chest

When the chest is notably asymmetrical, the following conditions
should be considered:

Congenital deformity
Congenital absence of the pectoralis major
Scoliosis
Intrathoracic disease—atelectasis, pleural effusion, air-containing
  cyst, etc.
Congenital asymmetry (hemihypertrophy, hemiatrophy)

Congenital absence of the pectoralis major is not rare. Simple
inspection together with awareness of the possibility will establish
the diagnosis. The condition may cause confusion in the x-ray of the
chest, by making one side of the chest appear to be more translucent
than the other. It may be combined with syndactyly (Poland's
syndrome).

Crying

All babies cry long before they laugh, and the causes of crying (or
laughing) are not always clear. I have discussed the subject in detail
elsewhere (Illingworth, 1955).

Many of the causes of crying are obvious. The usual ones are hunger, wind or any other discomfort. Some babies cry when the light is put out; others cry when the light is put on; all are likely to cry if the limbs or head are tightly held by one's hand.

One may summarise the causes of crying as follows:

A. Infants

(1) *Crying without disease*

Hunger due to fear of overfeeding. Thirst
Discomfort—wind, cold, heat, itching, evening colic, wet napkin, loud noises
Teething
Irritability on the breast
Personality
Crying on passing urine
Habit
Loneliness: desire to see surroundings, or to be picked up
Fatigue
Food forcing
Unexplained
Child abuse

(2) *Crying with disease*

Any infection
Headache, earache
Strangulated hernia
Intestinal obstruction and intussusception
Pink disease
Phenylketonuria
Coeliac disease
Autism

B. Older children (excessive crying only)

Personality
Insecurity
Habit
Hunger

Fatigue
Puberty
Early chorea
Any illness
Child abuse
Autism

The obvious cause of crying in an infant is hunger. A sensible mother feeds her young baby when he wants it, whether in the day or night. Rigid ideas about the feeding schedule, due to fears of causing 'bad habits', lead to a great deal of crying. Another rigid idea which leads to much crying from hunger is the fear of over-feeding. Many babies cry from hunger because someone is so ob-sessed by the fear of overfeeding them that they are half-starved. A baby's crying may be due to thirst, one cause of which is making the feeds with dried milk too strong (for instance, a heaped measure of milk powder in an ounce of water).

Discomfort from any cause may lead to crying. Excessive cold or excessive heat, pruritus (as from eczema), a wet napkin or a sudden loud noise, are all causes of crying.

Teething is a convenient condition to blame when a baby, six months or more of age, cries excessively, especially in the evening. It is reasonable to suggest that the eruption of a tooth through the periosteum may cause pain; but *much of the crying which is ascribed to teething is in fact related to habit formation in connection with sleep, due to parental mismanagement.* The usual age at which this sleep problem arises is nine to twelve months. The baby discovers that if he cries when put to bed he will be picked out of his cot and taken downstairs—and so he cries every time when put to bed. He may also discover that if he cries as soon as he awakens he will be picked up and taken either downstairs or into his parents' bed—and so he cries out every night. This crying is commonly ascribed by parents to 'indigestion', or 'awful wind', when in fact it is purely a habit which they have themselves caused.

Irritability and screaming in the newborn period when the baby is put to the breast is an annoying symptom, which leads to some babies being put on the bottle. Mavis Gunther (1955) ascribed it to the baby's nose becoming obstructed by his upper lip when feeding, or being blocked by the mother's breast tissue. It may be partly due to the mother trying to force the baby to suck, or fearing that the baby will bite her, withdrawing as soon as he begins to suck. In other cases it seems to be a feature of the baby's personality. The problem settles down within about ten days if patience is shown.

However wise the management, some babies cry excessively, and one can only ascribe it to the *personality*—which is largely inherited. Some babies seem to sense their mothers' anxiety and tenseness and cry as a result.

Babies commonly cry, often with a shriek, when *passing urine*. It is a normal feature, especially around the age of six months.

Many babies cry when left alone and are quiet when picked up. Many intelligent babies, from the age of six weeks or so, are not content to be left lying down with nothing to see. They are quiet when propped up so that they can see the fascinating activities of the kitchen.

In the weaning stage much crying is due to *efforts to force the child to take food*, especially food which he does not like. Rarely such crying may be due to food allergy.

It must be admitted that much crying in infants occurs without discoverable cause. If the crying continues when the child is picked up and fed, it must be assumed that it is due to some discomfort—perhaps *abdominal pain or headache*. Crying is usual when the baby feels tired.

Crying when the baby is unwell may be due to any *infection*, such as otitis media or pyelonephritis, or to intestinal obstruction (if there is also vomiting). One must always examine the *hernial orifices* for a strangulated hernia. The acute onset of screaming attacks should suggest the possibility of *intussusception*.

Pink disease should no longer occur, because mercury is no longer a constituent of teething powders, but one must remember the possibility of the mother having obtained a teething power from an old stock, or having applied an ointment containing mercury.

Crying is a feature of *phenylketonuria* until by proper treatment the serum phenylalanine level is reduced to normal. It follows that when there is unexplained crying the urine must be examined for phenylpyruvic acid. Crying is also a common feature of coeliac disease, until gluten is excluded.

In older children excessive crying may be a feature of the *personality*. It may be due to insecurity, and one must investigate the home and school background.

Crying at night is usually due to *habit formation*, the habit having continued from infancy. The child repeatedly cries out at night because he knows that his mother will come to him, perhaps read to him, play with him, give him a warm drink or take him into her own bed.

A child may cry because he is *hungry or tired*. Children at *puberty* commonly burst into tears with little or no provocation.

It is naturally important that when an older child is excessively lachrymose one must eliminate organic disease, such as *anaemia* or *pyelonephritis* or a persistent streptococcal throat infection.

When a child who previously behaved normally becomes unusually tearful, one must consider, in addition to the above, the possibility that he has early *chorea*. Emotional behaviour of this sort is a common early symptom. *Autism* is an occasional cause.

As in the case of the young infant, not all crying in the older child can be explained; but it is at least easier to find the cause in a child who is old enough to explain his feelings.

References

GUNTHER M. (1955) Instinct and the Nursing Couple. *Lancet*, **1**, 575.

ILLINGWORTH R.S. (1954) Three months' colic. *Arch. Dis. Childh.*, **29**, 165.

ILLINGWORTH R.S. (1955) Crying in infants and children. *Brit. med. J.*, **1**, 75.

Types of cry

There is an increasing interest in the nature of the cry of infants. Analysis of the cry by spectrographic methods has yielded interesting and useful information (Wasz-Hockert et al. 1963, Lind et al. 1965). Fisichelli and Karelitz (1963) showed that normal infants cry more rapidly after a stimulus than do children with brain abnormalities. It has long been known that babies with cerebral irritability, meningitis, hydrocephalus and kernicterus have a shrill, high pitched cry.

A hoarse gruff cry is characteristic of *hypothyroidism*.

The cat-like cry of the 'cri-du-chat' syndrome is also characteristic. This occurs in defective microcephalic infants. There is often some degree of hypertelorism, an antimongoloid slant of the eyes and low-set ears. It is associated with deletion of the distal portion of the short arm of one of the 4 to 5 chromosomes. The crying of the child with the *Cornelia de Lange syndrome* is said to sound like a bleating lamb.

The hoarseness of *laryngitis* is an obvious physical sign. More important is the presence of hoarseness in a child with stridor dating from birth (p. 147).

Other characteristic cries are the weak cry of the child with *amyotonia congenita* (or similar muscle weakness), and the whimper of the *seriously ill* child.

The child with pneumonia may have a grunting type of cry.

References

FISICHELLI V.R. & KARELITZ S. (1963) The cry latencies of normal infants and those with brain damage. *J. Pediat.*, **62**, 724.

KAJII T., HOMMA T., OIKAWA K., FURUYAMA M. & KAWARAZAKI T. (1966) Cri du chat syndrome. *Arch. Dis. Childh.*, **41**, 97.

LIND J., WASZ-HOCKERT O., VUORENKOSKI V. & VALENNE E. (1965) The vocalisation of a newborn brain damaged child. *Ann. Paediat. Fenniae*, **11**, 32.

MCARTHUR R.G. & EDWARDS J.H. (1967) De Lange syndrome. Report of 20 cases. *Can. Med. Ass. J.*, **96**, 1185.

WASZ-HOCKERT O., VALENNE E., VUORENKOSKI V., MICHELSSON K. & SOVIJARVI A. (1963) Analysis of some types of vocalisations in the newborn and in early infancy. *Ann. Paediat. Fenniae*, **9**, 1.

Insomnia

Refusal or failure to go to sleep is almost always a behaviour problem due to mismanagement, but because organic factors may be contributory, the subject will be briefly mentioned here.

The following are the main causes of defective sleep:

Mismanagement, including hunger
Evening colic (p. 97)
Mental subnormality

Vomiting, diarrhoea, polyuria, frequency of micturition.
Pruritus
In the older child—insecurity, fears, anxieties
Drugs

Mismanagement may consist of leaving the infant crying from hunger because of the fear that feeding a baby in the night will cause bad habits. Usually, however, sleep disturbance arising from mismanagement begins later in infancy, especially from about nine to fifteen months, when the child is allowed to discover that as soon as he cries (e.g. when put to bed, or on awakening), the mother will pick him up, take him downstairs, play with him, give him a warm drink or take him into her own bed (see crying, p. 241).

Some *mentally subnormal children* have an inverted sleep rhythm, sleeping by day and being wakeful by night.

Anything causing *vomiting, diarrhoea, polyuria* or *frequency of micturition* will cause sleep disturbance.

Pruritus, as from infantile eczema or scabies, may cause troublesome insomnia.

In the older child, *bad habit formation* beginning in infancy is the main cause of insomnia.

Other causes of sleep disturbance in the older child are *worries* and *anxieties about home or school,* or *fears of the dark* or *of shadows on the wall.*

Certain *drugs* may cause insomnia. They include amphetamine, diphenoxylate, ephedrine, griseofulvin, imipramine and vincristine. Fenfluramine may cause nightmares. Barbiturates or antihistamines may have a paradoxical effect and cause sleeplessness.

Diphenoxylate and imipramine are rare causes of sleep disturbance.

Reference

ILLINGWORTH R.S. (1972) *The Normal Child,* London, Churchill Livingstone, 5th Edn.

Mental subnormality

When one considers the obvious fact that approximately half the population has an I.Q. of less than 100, it is clear that backwardness is a common problem. Not all backwardness is due to a low level of intelligence, and many other conditions have to be kept in mind when one is considering the problem of a backward child.

The most common cause of backwardness in childhood is mental subnormality, and that condition will be considered first. I have discussed developmental diagnosis and the diagnosis of mental subnormality in detail elsewhere (Illingworth, 1972). Below is a summary of the main points in the diagnosis.

The first essential to the diagnosis of mental subnormality is a thorough knowledge of the normal and variations from the normal which do not amount to disease. One needs this knowledge in order to determine how far an infant has developed as compared with an average baby. One must also know the factors which may have affected his development, and know whether these factors will have a permanent effect or a reversible one. It is also useful to know about conditions which somewhat increase the likelihood that a child will be retarded—the factors which place him 'at risk' of mental subnormality.

One may summarise the factors which place him 'at risk' of mental subnormality as follows:

Family history of mental subnormality
Maternal rubella and possibly other virus infections in the first three
    months of pregnancy
Low birth weight, especially in relation to the duration of gestation
Maternal toxaemia, antepartum haemorrhage
Multiple pregnancy
Cerebral palsy
Congenital deformities

Convulsions in the newborn period, other than those due to hypo-
calcaemia
Hyperbilirubinaemia in the newborn period
Severe anoxia at birth, or cerebral haemorrhage

Factors which affect a child subsequently will be discussed in the
sections to follow.

One must not exaggerate the importance of any of these factors.
For instance, a mentally subnormal mother may give birth to a
normal child. Even a mongol woman may give birth to an
entirely normal infant. Maternal rubella in the first three months
affects the child in some 20 or 25 per cent of cases. Innumerable
low birth weight infants are mentally normal or superior. Maternal
toxaemia only slightly increases the risk of abnormality in the
foetus. Any major congenital deformity, such as a cleft palate or
congenital heart disease, slightly increases the risk of mental handicap. Many children who suffered severe anoxia at birth are mentally
and physically normal. Cerebral palsy, neonatal convulsions other
than those due to hypocalcaemia, and hyperbilirubinaemia (e.g.
serum bilirubin over 20 mgm per cent), significantly increase the
risk of a mental handicap.

It follows that one must take the history of any of the factors
above, but that one must not pay too much attention to them. One
bears them in mind and is alerted to the increased risk, but does not
exaggerate their importance. The next step (after the newborn
period) is to obtain a history of the milestones of development, so
that one can assess the rate of development from birth until the
present time.

The physical examination must include neurological examination
for signs of cerebral palsy and other conditions. The diagnosis of
mongolism and cretinism should be obvious. The examination must
include in particular a measurement of the maximum circumference
of the head, because the size of the head is governed largely by the
growth of the cranial contents. If the brain does not grow normally,
the head is usually small (p. 233). The head circumference of mentally subnormal infants is almost always small in relation to
their weight, unless they have hydrocephalus, megalencephaly or
hydranencephaly.

With regard to the developmental examination, it is essential to remember the all important principle that the mentally subnormal child is backward in all aspects of development, except occasionally in the motor field (sitting and walking). Hence the full term mentally subnormal baby at birth resembles a premature baby, in that he tends to sleep a large part of the day and night, he is apt to have difficulty in sucking and swallowing, he is apt to regurgitate and to fail to demand feeds. He is then late in passing the milestones of development. He is late in beginning to smile at his mother (average in normal full term infants—four to six weeks); he is late in following with his eyes and turning his head to sound (average three or four months), he is late in reaching out and grasping objects without their being placed in his hand (average five months), in chewing (average six or seven months), in helping his mother to dress him, by holding his arm out for a sleeve, in imitating byebye and playing patacake (all average 10 months), and later in speech. (The average child begins to combine words spontaneously at 21 to 24 months.) He is likely to be late in feeding himself with a cup without help (average 15 months) and in acquiring sphincter control (average 15 to 18 months for the first signs). Above all he shows less interest in his surroundings and concentrates badly, being easily distracted. He is also late in ceasing to take objects to the mouth, and in ceasing to cast objects to the ground, one after the other. (Average in both about 15 months.)

The diagnosis of mental subnormality is a most serious one to make, and it can only be made after careful consideration of the history, the child's development to date, the findings on examination, and an interpretation of the significance of each. It is wrong even to breathe a suspicion that the child is mentally defective until one is certain of one's ground, for it will cause the gravest distress and anxiety to the parents. I would strongly advise the family doctor to seek the opinion of an expert before imparting his diagnosis to the parents.

References

See p. 263.

Other causes of general backwardness

Many conditions other than mental subnormality may cause generalised backwardness in infancy and more especially in later childhood. For convenience I have listed them in three groups—factors in the child, in the home, in the teaching—though realising that there is some overlapping between these groups. I have discussed them in more detail elsewhere (Illingworth, 1972). They may be summarised as follows:

(a) Factors in the child

Delayed maturation: 'Slow starter'
Physical problems, such as cerebral palsy
Sensory problems—defective eyesight or hearing
Learning disorders
Personality—laziness, daydreaming, emotional blocks
Insecurity
The effect of failure
Poor concentration
Autism
Schizophrenia

(b) Factors in the home or environment

Emotional deprivation
Malnutrition (possibly)
Poor home—low expectation, poor example, etc.

(c) Factors in the teaching

Poor teaching
Lack of motivation
Absence from school
Changes from school to school
Special school instead of ordinary school

Factors in the child

Delayed maturation

Though delayed maturation is not as common as some parents imagine, it is a real entity. An infant may be retarded in all aspects of development and yet prove to be normal later. This could not be expected if there were microcephaly—and this fact alone indicates the importance of including a measurement of the maximum head circumference in the examination of every baby. The diagnosis of mental subnormality in infancy, unless it is severe, is difficult: the diagnosis of mental subnormality in an infant with a head of normal size in relation to weight is more than difficult—it is dangerous.

Delayed maturation is more frequent at school—the child doing badly in the subjects of the curriculum, and yet doing well later.

Physical problems

Cerebral palsy or muscular dystrophy may cause serious retardation apart altogether from the commonly accompanying mental subnormality. Amongst other things these conditions reduce the child's opportunity for learning.

Defective vision and hearing

When a child has poor eyesight or hearing from birth, he cannot know that he does not see or hear properly. It is the responsibility of others to make the diagnosis.

The diagnosis of defective vision is discussed on p. 159, and of defective hearing on p. 167.

Delayed reading

This is a major cause of backwardness at school.

The most common cause of delay in learning to read is mental subnormality, and this diagnosis must always be eliminated with the help of a psychologist before other causes, such as learning disorders, are considered.

A child may be delayed in learning to read as a result of bad environmental conditions, emotional deprivation or insecurity. He may be delayed by poor teaching, repeated or prolonged absence from school or by a visual or auditory defect, or poor concentration with overactivity. There is some relationship between delayed talking and reading with delay in the establishment of handedness.

Having eliminated the above factors, one should then consider the so-called 'learning disorders'.

Learning disorders

Learning disorders include dyslexia (difficulty in reading), dysphasia (difficulty in learning to speak), dysgraphia (difficulty in writing), and difficulties in spelling or spatial appreciation. Affected children are often clumsy in their movements. The difficulties commonly occur in combination. These children tend to leave too small or too large a space between written letters; they often write at an acute angle; they frequently reverse letters, such as *h* and *y*, *d* and *b*. They commonly read from right to left, and interpret, for instance, BUT as TUB, MEAT as MATE, SAW as WAS, transposing letters or syllables, and getting the order of the letters wrong. I saw a page of a boy's arithmetic book, with all the sums calculated like this:

$$16 + 1 = 71$$
$$13 + 1 = 41$$

Some of the children indulge in mirror writing. They may have inadequate auditory discrimination of speech sounds, interpreting, for instance, BUD as BUT, even though their actual hearing is normal. They may show an inability to synthesise into correct words letters which have individually been sounded correctly—interpreting, for instance, CLOCK as COCK. They fail to recognise or remember the shape of letters, however often they are told them, and confuse letters of similar shape. They may be able to spell out the word correctly but be unable to write it; they cannot correlate sound with the written word. Most of the children have difficulty in the establishment of handedness and in learning right-left differentiation. They are commonly ambidextrous or left-handed. They tend to read slowly and hesitantly, wriggling and distorting the face as they read. As they mature the concomitant signs and symptoms may disappear, leaving nothing but the reading difficulty. These difficulties often cause serious problems and embarrassment at school, often leading to behaviour problems such as truancy.

The correct diagnosis of dyslexia must be made only with the help of an educational psychologist. A proper I.Q. test must be carried out before the diagnosis can be established—and it is important that the diagnosis should be made, in order that the appropriate treatment can be arranged. This consists of combining the visual, auditory and kinaesthetic senses—the child being shown letters and words, hearing them and feeling them at the same time.

An important cause of dyslexia seems to be delay in maturation, some children being late in reading, just as others are late in walking or acquiring sphincter control. It is probable that in many cases there is a combination of factors. Those interested should read the papers by Ingram (1963, 1965).

The personality of the child has an important effect on his progress at school. Laziness is partly a personality problem, partly the effect of bad influence of others, and partly lack of interest in the work—which may be a matter of the child's lack of aptitude for a particular subject or the way in which the subject is taught. Daydreaming may interfere with school work. Sensitive children may develop emotional blocks to learning when they are afraid of the teacher or are being unduly hurried.

Insecurity is a most important cause of backwardness in intelligent children. The insecurity may be due to difficulties at home, to bullying at school or fear of a teacher. It has a powerful effect in lowering the standard of a child's work. *Failure* in work also has a bad effect on a child's progress. Success leads to success, and failure to a further lowering in the standard achieved.

Poor concentration

The most common cause of defective concentration is low intelligence—or an intelligence quotient below that of other members of the class.

Poor concentration may be due to daydreaming, to any source of insecurity, or to finding the work too easy. It may be due to boredom, dislike of the work, lack of motivation in the teaching or dislike of the teacher. It may be due to a defect of the eyesight or of hearing. Barbiturates or phenytoin are an important cause of defective concentration, either by causing drowsiness or by a more direct effect. Antiepileptic drugs may also act by causing folate deficiency, which can be corrected with consequent improvement in the child's performance. Fenfluramine and imipramine may be responsible for poor concentration. Frequent petit mal attacks may result in defective concentration.

Infantile autism

This is a serious condition in which the child from the earliest infancy shows no affection, preferring toys to persons. He has no desire to be picked up and cuddled when he is a baby. He may be poor at sucking, late in smiling, surprisingly undemanding if left alone and annoyed on being disturbed. He may fail to respond to the human voice while he responds to other sounds. His speech is seriously retarded. He may use words and intonate them well, but they bear no relation to the person listening to them and no relation to the existing situation. His head is of normal size and shape and he looks intelligent; yet he functions as a mentally defective child. He disregards his parents and tends to avert his gaze when spoken to. He is really an extreme introvert and isolates himself from the world. He may play with one toy in an obsessional way for hours, and is often especially fond of spinning toys: and he hates to change his occupation, having an intense desire for 'sameness'. He likes one particular routine, one particular toy or furniture arrangement and may develop a panic reaction if change occurs. He may adopt bizarre attitudes and postures.

When the diagnosis of autism is suspected, an expert should see the child.

Schizophrenia

The features of the schizophrenic child were discussed by a working party* in London, which suggested the following criteria for the diagnosis:

Gross and sustained impairment of emotional relationships with people: including aloofness, impersonal attitude to them, difficulty in mixing with other children.

* Working Party (1961) Schizophrenia in childhood. *Brit. Med. J.*, **2**, 890

Apparent unawareness of his own personal identity to a degree inappropriate to his age. Abnormal posturing, scrutiny of parts of the body. The confusion of personal pronouns.

Pathological preoccupation with particular objects or certain characteristics of them without regard to their accepted functions.

Sustained resistance to change in the environment and a striving to maintain or restore sameness.

Abnormal perceptual experience (in the absence of discernible organic abnormality), as implied by excessive, diminished or unpredictable response to sensory stimulants—for example, visual and auditory avoidance, insensibility to pain and temperature.

Acute excessive and seemingly illogical anxiety.

Speech may have been lost or never acquired, or may have failed to develop beyond a level appropriate to an earlier stage. There may be confusion of personal pronouns or mannerisms of use and diction. Though words or phrases may be uttered, they may convey no sense of communication.

Distortion in mobility patterns—excess (hyperkinesis), immobility (katatonia) or bizarre patterns—or ritualistic mannerisms such as rocking or spinning.

A background of serious retardation in which islets of normal, near normal or exceptional intellectual function or skill may appear.

Sometimes psychoses are superimposed on mental deficiency and this increases the difficulty of assessment.

Factors in the home

Factors in the home have a profound effect on the child's progress from infancy onwards. They include the home interests and example, the opportunities for the child to learn outside the home and school, praise for good work, expectation of success, and the right attitude to homework (implying that it is an understood thing that the homework will be done after the meal on returning from school). A poor home causes a considerable degree of retardation. Some parents actively discourage the child from doing his homework—or provide no place in which he can work away from the family and the television set.

Poor teaching

Backwardness may be due to poor teaching. Unless the teacher likes the child and the child the teacher, there are likely to be learning difficulties. Some teachers use the methods of threats, punishment, ridicule and sarcasm, instead of encouragement and praise, and then blame the child for not doing well. Lack of motivation is an important cause of backwardness: when a subject is badly taught and made uninteresting, the children are not likely to do well in it.

Prolonged absences from school are usually due to faulty management at home, but may be due to illness. Children are kept off school far too readily—and miss a great deal of education as a result. They are kept away from school for the most trivial cough or wheeze—and yet are taken shopping and attend the child welfare clinic with the baby brother. Frequent moves from school to school cause an emotional upheaval, and the child may find that work is being taught differently, or that he has missed much that has been taught. It has been shown that frequent short spells of absence from school cause more deterioration in performance than one long period of absence.

Some children are retarded by being sent to a special school instead of an ordinary school. The standard of education cannot be as high in a special school, where there is a wider scatter of age groups and intellectual levels in a class than in an ordinary school, and where less time is devoted to lessons.

For references, see p. 263.

Backwardness in individual fields of development

In considering individual fields of development one must always make due allowance for prematurity; e.g. if a baby were born two months prematurely, the average age for beginning to smile would be four to six weeks plus two months.

Smiling

All mentally subnormal and most autistic children are late in beginning to smile at the mother. A blind child will probably be late in beginning to smile.

Sitting and walking

The common causes of lateness in sitting and walking are:

Mental subnormality
Delayed motor maturation, usually familial
Hypertonia—cerebral palsy
Hypotonia
Muscular dystrophy
Emotional deprivation: institutional care
Lack of opportunity to sit and walk: illness
Excessive caution and timidity: dislike of bumps

By no means all mentally subnormal children are late in learning to sit and walk, but most are. A few mongols learn to sit at the usual age, but almost all are late in learning to walk.

When a child is late in sitting or walking, and no other abnormality can be found, it is common to find that the mother, father or sibling behaved in the same way. We presume that this is a matter of delayed maturation.

Cerebral palsy, particularly of the spastic and athetoid types, delays walking and in fact in severe cases may make it impossible. The hypotonias delay sitting and walking. A child with amyotonia congenita may never walk. Children with the more benign hypotonia may walk at five or six years of age. Some children with *muscular dystrophy* of the Duchenne type are late in learning to walk. This may be partly explained by a commonly associated slight mental subnormality, but the full explanation is not clear.

Children brought up in an institution are late in sitting and walking, partly because of emotional deprivation and partly because of lack of practice. If a child is kept on his back for prolonged periods, the age of sitting and walking is delayed.

Obesity almost certainly does not delay walking.

Many children refuse to walk without a hand held, long after they have become sufficiently mature to walk unaided.

Congenital subluxation of the hip does *not* delay walking. Many children are referred to orthopaedic surgeons on account of lateness in walking. This is irrational, and such children should be referred to the paediatrician.

Delayed sphincter control and enuresis

The following are the main causes of delayed control of the bladder:

Delayed maturation, usually a familial feature (primary enuresis)
Mental subnormality
Mismanagement of toilet training
Emotional deprivation
Organic causes
    Bladder-neck or urethral obstruction
    Ectopic ureter entering the vagina. Ureterocele
    Diverticulum of the anterior urethra
    Meningomyelocele
    Sacral agenesis
    Diastematomyelia
    Lipoma of the cauda equina
    Epispadias
    Ectopia vesicae
    Absent abdominal muscles with gross expansion of the posterior urethra
    Traumatic: after a circumcision operation
    Epilepsy

Many psychiatrists maintain that enuresis is entirely a psychological problem, while many paediatricians hold that there are two types of enuresis, primary and secondary, the primary kind being that in which the child has never been dry at night, and the secondary variety in which the child is dry for a period of months or years and then begins to wet the bed. They feel that the primary type has an organic basis in most cases, there being delay in maturation of the relevant part of the nervous system, some children being late in acquiring control of the bladder, just as others are late in learning to sit, walk or talk. In this variety there is usually a family history of the same complaint. If one of identical twins wets the bed, the other does; but if one of non-identical twins does, the likelihood of the other doing so is much less. No one would deny that psychological difficulties can be added to the problem of the child with primary enuresis. For instance, the mother is likely to smack the child for wetting his bed, may ridicule him or try to shame him for it—and so make him worse. In the same way, if she shows excessive anxiety about his toilet training, she is likely to cause emotional disturbance and add to his problem. I have discussed the problem in detail elsewhere (Illingworth, 1972).

The *mentally subnormal* child, being late in almost all aspects of development, is likely to be late in acquiring sphincter control.

Mismanagement of toilet training may cause delay in control of the bladder or relapse once control has been achieved. It may add psychological factors to the problem of delayed maturation. Mismanagement consists usually of excessively enthusiastic 'potting', compelling the child to sit on the pottie when he wants to get off and smacking him for not using it. Occasionally a parent does not give the child a chance to use the pottie when he wants it, and delays the acquisition of control. It is the usual thing for a mother to smack her child for wetting the bed—until she finds that it does not help, and then she merely scolds him.

A child brought up in an institution, or otherwise exposed to *emotional deprivation*, is likely to be late in acquiring control of the bladder.

The organic causes of urinary incontinence were fully reviewed in the article by Smith (1967). When a child has constant dribbling incontinence, day and night, bladder neck obstruction or urethral valves may be the cause in the boy, or an ectopic ureter or ureterocele in a girl. The older boy may dribble only after micturition, because some urine remains in the posterior urethra until the voluntary squeeze of the external urethral musculature relaxes, thus allowing the urine to dribble through. A diverticulum of the anterior urethra acts in the same way. The ectopic ureter in the girl may open into the urethra, or between the urethral and vaginal orifice, or near the hymen. In boy or girl, the diagnosis should immediately be suspected if there is dribbling incontinence. When the mother's story is equivocal, one should see that the child has a dry nappie on (if he still has one), and then observe when it becomes wet, by examining it every ten minutes or so.

The other organic causes, such as meningomyelocele, sacral agenesis, ectopia vesicae, absent abdominal muscles or lipoma involving the cauda equina, are obvious if looked for. The 'neurogenic bladder' is diagnosed by the dribbling of urine, the patulous anus, perineal anaesthesia, and the fact that urine can be expressed by firm suprapubic pressure. It is easy to miss the diagnosis of epispadias by failing to examine the penis. Diastematomyelia is less easy to diagnose. It may be associated with a meningomyelocele, or there may be a tuft of hair in the midline of the back which draws attention to the possibility of an underlying bone deformity. In addition to the incontinence there may be progressive weakness of the legs. The diagnosis is established by x-ray studies.

Incontinence following circumcision may be the result of putting a stitch through the urethra.

Bedwetting in the case of an epileptic child may be the result of a fit.

Secondary enuresis is usually due to psychological stress or insecurity. The cause may lie in worry at home or school, a move from house to house, a move to a new school or a spell in hospital. It is important to realise that when a child has recently acquired control of the bladder, anything causing frequency or polyuria is liable to cause enuresis. Hence in all cases one should examine the urine for sugar (i.e. for diabetes mellitus) and for the specific gravity (for renal failure and the other causes of polyuria). One must also examine a clean specimen under the microscope for excess of white cels and for organisms and culture it in order to eliminate a urinary tract infection.

Delayed speech

The following are the usual causes of delayed speech:

Mental subnormality
Delayed maturation, usually a familial trait
Emotional deprivation
Deafness
Twins
Psychoses—autism and schizophrenia (p. 253)
Aphasia
Unknown causes

The most common cause of delayed speech is *mental subnormality*. Probably all mentally subnormal children are late in learning to speak. Apart from this, the usual cause is delayed maturation: one nearly always finds that the mother, father or sibling was late in learning to speak.

A child brought up in an institution or otherwise subjected to *emotional deprivation* is likely to be late in learning to speak.

An important cause of delayed speech is *deafness*, which may be only for high tones. One must not be put off by the story that the child hears footsteps and many other noises. Suitable high tones for testing the child's hearing are the sounds PS, PHTH, and the crumpling of tissue paper, assuming that he cannot see the source of sound and that the source of sound is on a level with the ear and reasonably near (e.g. within one or two feet).

Twins are often late in speech—perhaps because the mother has less time to talk to twins than to singletons. The delay is unlikely to be due to the twins understanding each other without speaking properly.

Children with *infantile autism* or *schizophrenia* are late in speaking (p. 253).

Delayed speech is *not* due to laziness, it is *not* due to 'everything being done for him', it is *not* due to tongue tie, it is most unlikely to be due to jealousy.

There is some association between delayed speech and delay in the establishment of handedness. Whatever the cause parents and doctors should realise that a child fails to speak because he cannot speak. Adults tend to talk less to him, so that he hears less and is still further retarded.

Emotional causes include emotional deprivation, such as that due to institutional care, insecurity and worries. Poor teaching may be a cause. An undiagnosed visual defect may have led to the delay in reading.

We cannot always determine the cause of delayed speech. We do know that many children who are late in learning to speak are subsequently late in learning to read or write. When a child of three or four years of age is not saying any words and his hearing is known to be normal, and he is not autistic or mentally defective (i.e. has aphasia), the outlook is uncertain. All children with delayed speech development should be referred to an expert for diagnosis.

Dysarthria. In a child previously speaking normally, the sudden onset of dysarthria may be a premonitary symptom of *migraine*.

It may be a symptom of a wide variety of *degenerative diseases of the nervous system*, of cerebral tumour or congenital syphilis.

It may be due to certain *drugs*, namely diazepam, imipramine, phenytoin, primidone or sulthiame.

When a child has never spoken normally, dysarthria may be due to cerebral palsy, in which there is spasticity or incoordination of the muscles of speech, or to a cleft palate (or submucous cleft), structural abnormalities of the jaw, including malocclusion and macroglossia. Malpronunciation of the sounds m, n, ng, may be due to nasal obstruction. It has to be distinguished from dyslalia and severe lisp.

For references, see p. 263.

Mental deterioration

The usual causes of mental deterioration are as follows:

Emotional causes. Insecurity. Emotional deprivation
Poor teaching
Absences from school
Moves from school to school
Development of visual or auditory defects
Metabolic diseases
Severe hypoglycaemia, including insulin overdosage
Lead poisoning
Degenerative diseases of the nervous system
Cerebral tumour or abscess
Meningitis, encephalitis, cerebral thrombosis
Head injury
Effect of epilepsy
Drugs
Psychoses

Development of thyroid deficiency
Muscular dystrophy

At any age a child's progress may slow down as a result of *insecurity*, anxiety, worries or emotional deprivation. Laziness and loss of interest in the work in hand may also be important factors. In fact, insecurity in its broadest sense is one of the main causes of backwardness in intelligent children.

The question of *poor teaching*, *school absences* and *school moves* has already been discussed.

A child may develop a *defect of hearing or eyesight*, after having been previously normal, with the result that his school work deteriorates.

A variety of *metabolic diseases* leads to deterioration of a child's intelligence. They include particularly abnormalities of aminoacid metabolism, such as phenylketonuria, and of carbohydrate metabolism, such as galactosaemia; mucopolysaccharidoses; thyroid deficiency, hypercalcaemia and lipoidoses.

Severe hypoglycaemia, which is usually caused by insulin over-dosage, but which may arise spontaneously in association with fits, may lead to severe irreversible mental deficiency.

Lead poisoning causes serious mental deterioration. It must be remembered that mentally subnormal children are more likely to eat dirt or to take objects to the mouth than normal children, and so are more likely than others to develop lead poisoning—and so to deteriorate.

There are scores of *degenerative diseases of the nervous system*, mostly hereditary. They include in particular Friedreich's ataxia and Schilder's disease. Degenerative diseases of the nervous system are difficult to distinguish from an intracranial space-occupying lesion, and it follows that the necessary investigations should be carried out in hospital. They will include examination of the cerebrospinal fluid, x-ray of skull, echogram, air studies and perhaps marrow puncture.

Meningitis, encephalitis or head injury may cause serious mental subnormality in a previously normal child. Intracranial thrombosis as a result of dehydration or other causes may occur in infancy and have the same effect.

Epilepsy does not in itself cause serious mental deterioration, though epileptic fits may themselves be caused by the cerebral lesion which also causes mental deterioration. *Petit mal* is not usually associated with mental deterioration, though frequent attacks may cause a child in class to lose the thread of the discussion. Temporal lobe epilepsy is more likely than other forms of epilepsy to be associated with some deterioration. In infancy the so-called infantile spasms are almost invariably associated with mental deficiency and usually with deterioration. Major fits, if prolonged, may damage the brain by anoxia. Finally psychological problems associated with epilepsy may cause a child's school work to deteriorate.

Drugs given to an epileptic may have a retarding effect, leading to drowsiness, defective concentration and deterioration.

Psychoses such as schizophrenia cause serious deterioration in a child's performance.

Muscular dystrophy is commonly associated with some degree of mental deterioration.

References

ARTHUR L.J.H. (1965) Some hereditary syndromes that include deafness. *Develop. Med. Child. Neurol.*, **7**, 395.

CLANCY H. & McBRIDE G. (1969) The autistic process and its treatment. *J. Child Psychol. Psychiat.*, **10**, 233.

DALE, R.R. & GRIFFITH S. (1965) *Downstream*, London, Routledge and Kegan Paul. (Backward intelligent children.)

HERMANN, K. (1959) *Reading Disability*, Copenhagen, Munksgaard.

ILLINGWORTH R.S. (1968) How to help a child to achieve his best. *J. Pediat.*, **73**, 61.

ILLINGWORTH R.S. (1965) *The Normal School Child: His Problems Physical and Emotional*, London, Heinemann.

ILLINGWORTH R.S. (1972) *Development of the Infant and Young Child, Normal and Abnormal*, Edinburgh, Churchill Livingstone, 5th Edn.

INGRAM T.T.S. (1963) Delayed development of speech with special reference to dyslexia. *Proc. Roy. Soc. Med.*, **56**, 199.

INGRAM T.T.S. & MASON A.W. (1965) Reading and writing difficulties in childhood. *Brit. med. J.*, **2**, 463.

LUCAS A.R., RODIN E.A. & SIMSON C.B. (1965) Neurological assessment of children with early school problems. *Develop. Med. Child. Neurol.*, **7**, 145.

MORLEY M.E. (1972) *The Development and Disorders of Speech in Childhood*. Edinburgh, Livingstone.

Neubauer C. (1970) Mental deterioration in epilepsy due to folate deficiency. *Brit. med. J.,* 2, 759.

Schechter M.D. (1971) Dyslexia. *Australian Paediat. J.,* 7, 123.

Smith E.D. (1967) Diagnosis and management of the child with wetting. *Australian Paediat. J.,* 3, 193.

Zangwill O.L. (1968) Language and Language Disorders. In Dorfman P., *Child Care in Health and Disease.* Chicago, Year Book Publishers.

Thirst

Young babies (and mentally subnormal children) may not show thirst, and may become dehydrated as a result. Babies, for instance, with nephrogenic diabetes insipidus have to be forced to take more fluid than they demand, but have polydipsia when older. Some normal young children with fever due to infection may not demand sufficient fluid and have to be persuaded to take more.

Thirst is likely to result in older children from excessive perspiration due to a high outside temperature, over-clothing or fever. It may be due to anything causing polyuria, such as diabetes insipidus, diabetes mellitus, chronic renal disease, hypercalcaemia and renal acidosis.

Polydipsia and thirst may be a habit, and commonly are so. It is not easy to distinguish habit polydipsia from that due to diabetes insipidus, and admission to hospital is necessary for the purpose of investigation (see Polyuria, p. 267).

Rare causes of polydipsia include phaeochromocytoma or neuroblastoma.

The diagnosis of a urinary tract infection

A urinary tract infection is difficult to diagnose with certainty in general practice (and there are often difficulties in making the diagnosis in hospital). Mistakes are commonly made in two directions: the diagnosis is made when there is in fact no urinary infection, and it is missed when there is an infection. The reasons for the mistakes are varied. Many regard scalding on micturition or frequency as definitely indicating an infection, and regard these symptoms as necessary before making the diagnosis. Both of these beliefs are incorrect. Discomfort on micturition may be due to a meatal ulcer or balanitis in the boy, or soreness of the vulval region, as in a nappie rash, in the girl. There are many other causes of frequency (p. 267). These symptoms in fact are the exception rather than the rule in a urinary tract infection. In an acute infection the common symptoms are fever, vomiting, rigors, meningism and febrile convulsions (under the age of five). There may be abdominal discomfort and sometimes diarrhoea. There is unlikely to be tenderness in the loin. Another common misbelief is the idea that there must be albumin in the urine or that the presence of albumin confirms the diagnosis. In fact albumin is present in less than half of all cases. Frank haematuria is definitely unusual. In a chronic urinary tract infection the only symptoms are commonly lack of energy, poor appetite and other vague symptoms which do not point to the urinary tract.

The chief difficulty in practice lies in obtaining a clean non-contaminated specimen (in a girl) and in getting the specimen promptly to the laboratory for culture. A catheter specimen should not be taken because of the risk of introducing an infection. In order to obtain a clean specimen from a girl after infancy, she should squat or crouch if possible over a sterile bowl. The labia should be separated and swabbed with sterile normal saline in the direction of the anus. The labia should be held apart when the child is micturating. In order to obtain a clean specimen from a boy the prepuce is retracted if possible and the glans is swabbed with sterile normal saline. The child is asked to micturate while the prepuce is held retracted. From either a boy or girl a midstream specimen is obtained if possible by interposing a sterile container or a dipslide in the stream of urine just after micturition has started. The dipslide is coated with a bacteriological medium. Immediately after the urine has covered it, the slide is inserted into the sterile bottle supplied and is subsequently sent to the laboratory. The Uriglox test has not proved to be reliable.

When the child is too young to micturate on request, a plastic bag is attached to him (or her). A satisfactory one is the Chironseal urine collector, devised at the Hospital for Sick Children, Great

Ormond Street, London. When it is still uncertain whether the urine has been contaminated, the paediatrician may carry out a bladder puncture in order to establish the diagnosis.

If there is delay in getting the urine to the laboratory, the result will be valueless, however carefully it has been collected. In spite of all precautions contamination is still liable to occur, and one should never rely on a single specimen for diagnosis or exclusion of a urinary tract infection. The diagnosis should always be confirmed by a second specimen.

Microscopy of a noncentrifuged specimen will show an excess of white cells and the presence of organisms in severe infections, but this cannot be relied on to eliminate the diagnosis, which can only be made in the laboratory, where a centrifuged specimen will be examined for the presence of an excess of white cells, and where a culture of the urine can be made, with a total viable count and sensitivity studies, so that the correct drug can be prescribed. It is most important to realise that urinary tract infections may be shown by bacteriuria, as shown by the total viable count on culture, *without pyuria*. A total viable count of 100,000 organisms or more is accepted as indicating infection, especially if there is a pure growth. A count of 10,000 should lead to the testing of a further specimen. A *severe* infection can be detected by the family doctor without a microscope if the urine remains turbid after boiling and after adding acetic acid, provided that there is no blood in the urine. The urine infected by *E. coli* may have a 'fishy' smell. It is definitely only the severe infections which can be detected in this way. Hence *a child suspected of having a urinary tract infection should be referred to a hospital outpatient department*. This will avoid treating those who have no infection, giving the wrong treatment to those who have, and failing to diagnose important urinary tract anomalies which can only be detected by pyelography. One may add that the effectiveness of treatment has to be checked repeatedly by culture of clean specimens, during and after the administration of the drug. This is carried out in hospital.

References

See p. 274.

Frequency of micturition and polyuria

The common causes to consider are the following:

The normal frequency in a toddler

Attention-seeking device

Any cause of polyuria—polydipsia, diabetes mellitus, diabetes insipidus, hypercalcaemia, renal failure, salt-losing type of adrenocortical hyperplasia, Conn's syndrome

Pelvic appendicitis

Nephritis

Urinary tract infection.

Drugs

A toddler who is learning control of the bladder always has urgency and cannot wait once he feels the desire to pass urine. In children with enuresis of the primary type this urgency commonly continues for some years, sometimes into adult life. A toddler may in addition develop what appears to the mother to be frequency of micturition, when it is in reality an attention-seeking device. The child discovers that as soon as he demands to pass urine his mother drops everything and rushes him to the pottie; he then demands to pass urine every few minutes, and his mother in her anxiety to train him does not realise the true nature of the frequency.

Frequency may be the result of a *urinary tract infection*, but it is not a common symptom of that condition. It may also result from anything causing *polyuria. Conn's syndrome*, which is rare, includes polyuria, polydipsia, alkalosis, hypokalaemia, hypertension, albuminuria and a urine of low specific gravity.

The essential preliminary investigations include the testing for sugar and for a fixed low specific gravity.

When an older child has polyuria not due to diabetes mellitus it is essential to distinguish *polyuria of psychogenic origin*, due to habit polydipsia, from diabetes insipidus. This requires considerable laboratory facilities, including examination for the serum osmolarity, which is low or normal in psychogenic types, and raised in diabetes insipidus. If pitressin is given and causes a more concentrated urine than restriction of fluid alone, there is good evidence of diabetes insipidus of pituitary type. If it does not produce a more concentrated urine the diagnosis is likely to be compulsive polydipsia.

Frequency of micturition may result from a *pelvic appendicitis*. It may also occur in *acute nephritis*—even though in fact the total urinary output is reduced.

Drugs which may cause frequency and polyuria include antihistamines and Vitamin D excess.

References

See p. 274.

Scalding on micturition: dysuria

It is normal for a baby in the first few months to scream on micturition. Some scalding on micturition may be due merely to the urine being concentrated as the result of a raised temperature in an infection.

When an older child complains of discomfort on micturition, a local examination of the genital area should be carried out. A common cause is ammonia dermatitis, a meatal ulcer or soreness of the vulva. It could result from mephonamide crystalluria.

Dysuria may be caused by a urinary tract infection. Acute nephritis may be accompanied by pain on micturition with some frequency.

It is a serious mistake to treat a child as a urinary tract infection on the basis of symptoms without establishing the diagnosis in the laboratory.

References

See p. 274.

Haematuria

When considering the causes of haematuria, it is convenient to consider the following conditions:

Blood diseases
Miscellaneous general diseases—glandular fever, scurvy, collagen diseases
Drugs
Trauma

Conditions in the kidney

  Inflammation—nephritis, pyelonephritis, tuberculosis
  Tumours: Wilms's tumour, polycystic kidney
  Calculi, crystalluria
  Renal vein thrombosis
  Hydronephrosis
  Schistosomiasis
  Infarction
  Angioma

Conditions in the ureter
Conditions in the bladder
Conditions in the urethra
Effect of exertion
Unexplained

Blood diseases which cause haematuria include haemophilia, sickle cell anaemia, thrombocytopenic purpura and leukaemia. Haematuria commonly follows Henoch-Schönlein purpura, as a result of a complicating nephritis. Scurvy, glandular fever and the collagen diseases are occasionally accompanied by haematuria.

Certain *drugs* cause haematuria. The main ones are sulphadiazine or certain other members of the sulphonamide group. The crystals can be found on microscopy of the urine. Other drugs causing haematuria include acetazolamide, aminophylline, bacitracin, cyclophosphamide, kanamycin, P.A.S., phensuccimide, phenytoin, troxidone.

The possibility of *injury* to the kidney must be remembered.

Acute nephritis is the commonest cause of haematuria in a child. The symptoms may be severe, including headache, vomiting, fits and puffy eyes, but symptoms may be almost absent, without visible oedema. The diagnosis would be established by finding albumin, red blood cells and granular and cellular casts in the urine. In acute nephritis the ESR is always raised. This is a useful non-specific test when one is uncertain whether the child has nephritis or not because some of the commonly found features, such as elevation of the blood pressure or blood urea, are missing.

Naked eye haematuria may occur in *pyelonephritis*, but is unusual. Haemorrhagic cystitis may result from an *adenovirus* infection or from *cyclophosphamide*.

Tuberculosis of the kidney is now rare in Britain. The tuberculin test will be positive. The diagnosis is confirmed by the finding of sterile pyuria, detection of tubercle bacilli in the centrifuged deposit, and isolation of the tubercle bacillus on culture or guinea pig inoculation.

Tumours and cysts of the kidney include the nephroblastoma (Wilms's tumour), polycystic disease and angioma of the renal pelvis. Wilms's tumour occurs particularly in the first four years. The initial complaint is usually an abdominal mass, but haematuria may occur. Diagnosis is made by pyelography and sometimes by laparotomy.

Renal calculi are rare in children unless they are confined to bed for prolonged periods with orthopaedic conditions.

Renal vein thrombosis occurs mainly in the first few months of life, commonly following an infection elsewhere. The diagnosis is suspected when a child suddenly develops haematuria, a renal mass and perhaps oedema. *Infarction of the kidney* may occur in subacute bacterial endocarditis.

Conditions in the bladder include polypi, diverticula and foreign bodies. The latter should never be forgotten in a girl. I have seen a child admitted to hospital on ten occasions on account of haematuria, before a safety pin was found in the bladder. Polypi and diverticula are diagnosed by cystograms and cystoscopy.

Bleeding may arise from a *urethral caruncle* in a girl or a *meatal ulcer* in a boy. The blood in such a case would be seen at the end of micturition.

In an occasional child haematuria follows *exertion* (Illingworth and Holt, 1957).

After the most complete investigation, including renal biopsy, it may be impossible to determine the cause of the haematuria.

For conditions causing a colour change in the urine suggestive of haematuria, see p. 272.

References

See p. 274.

Changes in the colour of the urine

The following conditions are associated with unusual colouration of the urine:

Dark colour
  Concentration, as in fever
Dark yellow
  Bile
  Carotene-containing foods
Red
  Haemoglobinuria
  Favism
  Infection of baby's alimentary tract by serrata marcescens
  Rhodamine B in foodstuffs
  Blackcurrant juice, blackberries, rose hip syrup
  Beeturia
  Drugs
Red brown
  Urates
  Porphyria
  Myoglobinuria

Dark brown or black
  Alkaptonuria
  Tyrosinosis
  Melanosis
Yellow
  Bile
  Carotene-containing foods
Blue
  Hypercalcaemia

Bile—is demonstrated by the Fouchet test.

Haemoglobinuria occurs when there is rapid haemolysis.

The red colour of the urine in *beeturia* is due to the pigment betanin in the beet. The red colour changes to yellow when alkali is added, and returns to red on acidification.
Urates disappear on boiling.
In porphyria, the urine may be normal in colour when passed, but changes to Burgundy red on exposure to light. There may be haemolytic anaemia, photosensitivity and hypertrichosis.
The urine in myoglobinuria is red brown and gives a positive benzidine or guaiac test. It follows crush injuries, electric shocks, severe exercise or other causes. There may be muscle pains, chills and vomiting. The diagnosis is confirmed by spectroscopy and paper electrophoresis of the urine.
In alcaptonuria the urine becomes dark on standing. The nappie may show a black stain. The urine gives a colour change with Benedict's reagent and ferric chloride gives a fleeting blue colour.

Some drugs, other than those mentioned in the table on p. 273, may colour the urine red or red brown. They include rifampicin, sulphonamides, quinine and pamaquin.

The table on p. 273, reproduced with permission from Shirkey's excellent book *Pediatric Therapy* (1968), summarises the colour changes which may result from drugs.

References

BOROIAN T.V. & ATTWOOD C.R. (1965) Myoglobinuria. *J. Pediat.,* **67,** 69.
Brit. Med. J. (1963) Annotation. Beeturia, **2,** 948.

Drugs that colour the urine

...ne colour	Associated drug or chemical	Urine colour	Associated drug or chemical
	Methylene blue	Pink and red to red brown —cont'd	Emodin (alkaline urine)
...rn to ...ck	Aniline dyes		Eosins (red with green fluorescence)
	Cascara		Hematuria producers (mercuric salts, irritants, etc.)
	Chlorinated hydrocarbons		Hemolysis producers
	Hydroxyquinone		Phenindione (Danilone, Hedulin, Indon)
	Melanin		Phenolic metabolites (glucuronides)
	Methocarbamol (Robaxin)		Phenolphthalein (alkaline urine)
	Naphthalene		
	Naphthol		Phensuximide (Milontin)
	Nitrites		Porphyrins
	Phenol		Prochlorperazine (Compazine)
	Phenyl salicylate (salol)		
	Pyrogallol		Santonin (alkaline urine)
	Quinine		Thiazolsulfone (Promizole)
	Resorcinol (resorcin)		Urates (especially newborn infants and during tumour lysis)
	Rhubarb		
	Santonin		
	Senna		
	Thymol		
...en (blue ...us yellow)	Anthraquinone		
	Arbutin	Rust	Chlorzoxazone (Paraflex)
	Bile pigments		
	Eosins	Yellow or brownish	Danthrone (Dorbane) (acid urine)
	Methocarbamol (Robaxin)		Heavy metals (bismuth mercury)
	Methylene blue		Liver poisons (jaundice)
	Resorcinol (resorcin)		Alcohol
	Tetrahydronaphthalene		Arsenicals
	Thymol		Carbon tetrachloride
...enta to ...rple	Fuchsin		Chloral hydrate
	Phenolphthalein		Chlorinated hydrocarbon
			Chlorobutanol (chlorbutol, Chloretone)
...nge to ...ange red	Phenylazopyridine (Pyridium)		Chloroform
			Cinchophen
...nge to ...d brown	Combinations of phenylazopyridine (Pyridium) and other drugs used as urinary antiseptics; many of the trade names begin with *azo*		Naphthalene
			Neocinchophen
			Nitrofurantoins
			Pamaquine (Aminoquin, Beprochine, Gamefar, Plasmoquine, Praequine Quipenyl)
	Santonin		Sulfonamides
...k and red ...red brown	Aminopyrine		Tribromoethanol with amylene hydrate (Avertin)
	Anthraquinine and its dyes		
	Antipyrine (Pyrazoline)	Yellow or green	Carotene-containing foods
	Chrysarobin (alkaline urine)		Methylene blue
	Cinchophen		Riboflavin
	Danthron (Dorbane) (pink to violet—alkaline urine)		Vitamin B complex
	Diphenylhydantoin (Dilantin)		Yeast concentrate

Cone T.E. (1968) Diagnosis and treatment—some syndromes, diseases and conditions associated with abnormal coloration of the urine or diaper. *Pediatrics*, **41**, 654.

Conn J.W. (1955) Primary aldosteronism. *J. Lab. clin. Ped.*, **45**, 3.

Dies F., Rangel S. & Rivera A. (1961) Differential diagnosis between diabetes insipidus and compulsive polydipsia. *Ann. intern. Med.*, **54**, 710.

Drug and Therapeutics Bulletin (1972) Uriglox test for asymptomatic bacteriuria. **10**, 35.

Glasgow E.F., Moncrieff M.W. & White R.H.R. (1970) Symptomless haematuria in childhood. *Brit. med. J.*, **2**, 687.

Illingworth R.S. & Holt K.S. (1951) Transient rash and haematuria after exercise and emotion. *Arch. Dis. Childh.*, **32**, 254.

Illingworth R.S. (1972) *The Normal Child*, London, Churchill Livingstone, 5th Edn.

Lancet (1963) Annotation. Establishing the cause of Polyuria, **2**, 821.

McFarland J.B. (1965) Renal vein thrombosis. *Quart. J. Med.*, **34**, 269.

Numazaki Y., Shigeta S., Kumasaka T., Miyazawa T., Yamanaka M., Yano N., Tayai S. & Ishida N. (1968) Acute haemorrhagic cystitis in children. *New Engl. J. Med.*, **278**, 700.

Pyles C.V. & Eliot C.R. (1965) Pyuria and bacteriuria in infants and children. *Am. J. Dis. Child.*, **110**, 628.

Shirkey H.C. (1968) Pediatric Therapy. Mosby, St. Louis.

Tunnessen W.W., Smith C. & Oski F.A. (1969) Beeturia. *Am. J. Dis. Child.*, **117**, 424.

Oedema

Face

Oedema of the face may be caused by the following conditions:

General disease—haemolytic disease (in the newborn baby), nephritis, heart failure, trichiniasis
Rubbing the eyes excessively; crying
Angioneurotic oedema
Drugs
Acute antrum infection, infection around the face
Cavernous sinus thrombosis
Melkersson's syndrome
Dermatomyositis
Infectious mononucleosis

Oedema which appears to be confined to the face may be part of generalised oedema.

Excessive *rubbing of the eyes*, commonly due to itching of the eyes, as in hayfever, may cause periorbital oedema.

Angioneurotic oedema may be due to a variety of allergens. There is a rare congenital form.

Drugs may cause oedema of the face. By far the commonest is aspirin; others include amitriptyline, cephaloridine, chlordiazepoxide, demethylchlortetracyline (ledermycin), indomethacin, methimazole, nitrofurantoin, nortriptyline, penicillin, primidone, troxidone.

Oedema of the face may be caused by *infections in the vicinity* such as an acute antrum infection, a boil, dental abscess, orbital cellulitis, osteitis or cavernous sinus thrombosis.

Oedema of the eyelids may be due to *dermatomyositis or infectious mononucleosis*.

Arm

Oedema of the arm of a newborn baby may be due to an arm presentation.

A mother may be greatly alarmed when she picks up a baby from his bed in the morning and finds that one arm is swollen, cold and blue. There is pitting oedema. This is due not to the child lying on the affected arm, but to the arm having become uncovered when the temperature of the room is low. In a few hours the oedema disappears and the arm becomes normal in colour and appearance.

Legs

Congenital asymmetry may be confused at first with oedema. In this condition one half of the body is larger than the other, but there is no oedema.

Unilateral limb enlargement from birth may be due to a *lymphangioma or arteriovenous abnormality*, but there is not usually oedema. If the oedema is unilateral, and dates from birth, Milroy's oedema should be considered. This is largely lymphatic and there is little pitting.

Oedema of both legs in a girl, or in a boy in whom the testes cannot be palpated, suggests *Turner's syndrome*. Chromosome examination should be carried out.

Oedema of both legs may result from *ascites*.

Sickle cell anaemia may cause oedema of the limbs.

Oedema may be due to compression stenosis of the left common iliac vein by an overriding right common iliac artery ('iliac compression syndrome', Cockett *et al.*, 1967).

Genitalia

Oedema of the genitalia is common in normal newborn infants.

Oedema of the scrotum may be caused by an insect bite or sensitivity to detergents used for washing the nappies or pants. Sometimes the cause of recurrent short attacks of oedema of the scrotum cannot be determined.

Oedema of the scrotum has to be distinguished from epididymitis (in which there would be marked tenderness), swelling around a pustule, torsion of the testis (p. 107) and rupture of the urethra with extravasation of urine.

Lower part of body

This may be due to an adherent pericardium or obstruction of the inferior vena cava.

Sternum

This occurs at the onset of mumps.

Generalised oedema

In the newborn baby, the common causes of oedema are as follows:
Immaturity of the kidney
Haemolytic disease
Maternal diabetes

After the newborn period, the causes of oedema are mainly the following:

(i) Hypoproteinaemia

    Defective protein intake, kwashiorkor, beriberi

    Nephritis and the nephrotic syndrome

    Fibrocystic disease of the pancreas; steatorrhoea

    Protein loss in association with burns, eczema or severe suppuration

    Diarrhoea

    Liver disease; galactosaemia, cirrhosis

    Protein-losing enteropathy

    Unexplained

(ii) Heart failure

(iii) Increased capillary permeability

    Anaemia

    Henoch-Schönlein purpura

    Aspirin sensitivity

    Angioneurotic oedema

(iv) Excessive intake of sodium or fluid

    Excessive infusion

    Hyperelectrolytaemia due to faulty infant feeding

(v) Diabetes mellitus, on instituting treatment

This classification is not entirely accurate, but it serves as a guide.

Oedema without albuminuria may be the presenting symptom in *fibrocystic disease of the pancreas*.

Severe *burns, exudative eczema, suppuration or severe chronic diarrhoea* leads to protein loss and oedema.

Generalised oedema may be the result of *liver disease*, such as cirrhosis of the liver or galactosaemia.

Protein-losing enteropathy is a condition in which there is an excessive loss of protein in the stools without diarrhoea.

There remains a group of cases in which there is temporary oedema with hypoproteinaemia without discoverable cause.

It should be noted that the facial oedema in children with the *nephrotic syndrome* (or other cause of oedema) may be asymmetrical in distribution, owing to the child lying on one side in sleep.

Generalised oedema due to *heart failure* is rare in children. The diagnosis will not necessarily be obvious. There may be a murmur or cyanosis pointing to congenital heart disease, but heart failure may occur without a murmur in paroxysmal tachycardia, coarctation of the aorta, Fallot's tetralogy (in early infancy), transposition of the vessels or anomalous venous drainage, and when heart failure develops the murmur of a patent ductus or of a ventricular septal defect may disappear. Heart failure may also occur without a murmur in myocarditis, fibroelastosis or severe anaemia.

Aspirin sensitivity may manifest itself by generalised oedema.

A variety of allergic causes may be responsible for angioneurotic oedema, but it is not normally easy to detect the allergen.

Excessive sodium or fluid intake is usually due to an excessive intravenous infusion. Faulty feeding may result in oedema in premature infants; too concentrated a formula may lead to oedema by causing hypernatraemia.

Slight oedema lasting for a few days occurs in some ten per cent of children when treatment of *diabetes mellitus* is commenced (Klein *et al.*, 1962).

References

Cockett F.B., Thomas M.L. & Negus D. (1967) Iliac vein compression—its relation to ileofemoral thrombosis and the post-thrombotic syndrome. *Brit. med. J.*, **2**, 14.

Cochran W. (1970) Severe dermatitis and biological detergents. *Brit. med. J.*, **2**, 362.

Donaldson V.H. & Rosen F.S. (1966) Hereditary angio-neurotic oedema. *Pediatrics*, **37**, 1017.

Fisher D.A. (1966) Obscure and unusual edema. *Pediatrics*, **37**, 506.

Gordon R.S. (1961) Protein losing enteropathy in the sprue syndrome. *Lancet*, **1**, 55.

Illingworth R.S. & Finch E. (1954) Chronic generalised oedema and hypoproteinaemia of unknown origin. *Arch. Dis. Childh.*, **29**, 507.

Illingworth R.S. & Finch E. (1954) Temporary generalised oedema of obscure origin. *Arch. Dis. Childh.*, **29**, 513.

Klein R., Marks J.F., Roldan E., Sherman F.E. & Fetterman G.H. (1962) The occurrence of peripheral oedema and subcutaneous glycogen deposition following the initial treatment of diabetes mellitus in children. *J. Pediat.*, **60**, 87.

Kundstater R.H. (1965) Melkersson's syndrome. *Am. J. Dis. Child.*, **110**, 559.

Pittman F.E., Harris R.C. & Barker H.G. (1964) Transient edema and hypo-proteinemia. *Am. J. Dis. Child.*, **108**, 189.
Sacrez R., Geisert J., Willard D., Lahlou B. & Peter M.O. (1970) Precocious oedema in newborn infants. *Rev. Pédiatrie*, **6**, 203.

Delayed puberty in the girl and primary amenorrhoea

By the term delayed puberty I mean absence of menstruation by the age of sixteen. By primary amenorrhoea I mean the absence of menstruation; by secondary amenorrhoea I mean amenorrhoea after one or more menstrual periods.

Delayed puberty is due to the following conditions:

Normal variation
Familial factors
Severe malnutrition, including steatorrhoea
Congenital heart disease and other chronic illnesses
Thyroid deficiency (possible)

Primary amenorrhoea is due to the following causes:
Turner's syndrome and other forms of gonadal dysgenesis
Pituitary dwarfism
Gonadotrophin deficiency
Absence of the vagina or uterus
Haematocolpos
Ovarian cyst or tumour
Adrenocortical hyperplasia
Testicular feminisation syndrome

There may be *unexplained variations* in the age of puberty without a family history of the same condition and without discoverable cause. Malnutrition or any severe chronic illness may delay the onset of puberty. Girls of small build are likely to reach puberty later than those of big build.

When there is no sign of puberty by the age of 16, and there is no relevant family history, full examination and investigation is required in order to eliminate the causes of primary amenorrhoea.

Pituitary dwarfism may be unexplained, or be due to a pituitary tumour (craniopharyngioma or chromophobe adenoma). The child is dwarfed but has normal proportions. There are usually no secondary sexual characteristics. Investigations necessary include X-ray of the skull for the pituitary fossa and tests of pituitary function including the secondary effects on the thyroid and adrenal.

Gonadotrophin deficiency may be congenital. Affected children may be tall. The diagnosis is made by absence of secondary sexual characteristics and by the estimation of the urinary gonadotrophins.

Anatomical causes of amenorrhoea should be found on physical examination. The diagnosis may be suggested by the absence of menstruation in the presence of normal sexual characteristics. *Haematocolpos* should be found by examination of the vaginal introitus. *Adrenocortical hyperplasia* would be diagnosed by the virilisation, short stature at the normal age of puberty, the enlarged clitoris and the urinary 17 ketosteroid estimation.

The testicular feminisation syndrome is characterised by a normal female appearance with normal or increased height and full breast development with pale areolae. There is little or no body hair, pubic or axillary. There is commonly a family history of amenorrhoea. The gonads may be intraabdominal or in an inguinal hernia. On rectal examination no uterus can be palpated. The buccal smear is chromatin negative.

It will be seen that the presence of normal pubic hair, normal breast development and normal looking genitalia in general implies less serious conditions; that shortness of stature suggests Turner's syndrome or pituitary disease, and that normal physical growth suggests that there is no disease of the pituitary.

Investigations necessary include the buccal smear, chromosome studies, estimation of urinary oestrogens, gonadotrophins or 17 ketosteroids and examination of the urinary sediment or vaginal smear for oestrogenisation. It may be necessary to carry out tests for pituitary function including the metyrapone test, and for secondary effects on the thyroid (protein-bound-iodine) and adrenal. In certain circumstances a laparotomy may be required.

References

See p. 287.

Some other gynaecological problems

Secondary amenorrhoea and irregular menstruation

It is usual for menstruation to be irregular or scanty for several months after the first period has occurred. It is normal for a year or more to elapse between the first and second period, and for six months to elapse between periods in the second year (McArthur, Truman and Connolly, 1964). Approximately 40 periods occur before the regular adult pattern is established.

Amenorrhoea commonly occurs during the summer, or when there is emotional stress as on starting at a new school. It may occur when weight is being reduced on account of obesity or in malnutrition.

Pregnancy must always be considered when amenorrhoea develops.

Vaginal bleeding

A small amount of vaginal bleeding in the girl between the age of five and ten days is normal. It is due to maternal oestrogens and is not related to haemorrhagic disease of the newborn.

Vaginal bleeding at any subsequent age, without associated signs of puberty, should raise the possibility of trauma, foreign body or possibly a tumour. It may also occur as a result of a blood disease. The blood may arise from the vulva, vagina or uterus. The blood may have come from the urethra.

Vaginal bleeding may be the first indication of sexual precocity.

It is said that ethosuccimide can cause vaginal bleeding.

It is essential that vaginal bleeding before the age of puberty should be investigated because of the importance of possible causes.

Vaginal discharge

It is normal for the newborn girl in the first few days to have a thin vaginal discharge, and between the fifth and the tenth day some bleeding may occur.

After infancy a clear mucoid discharge is common and of no significance. Unless it is offensive or purulent it should be ignored. It may be due to lack of cleanliness, to eczema, ammonia dermatitis, or to mild itching leading to rubbing. A small girl playing in a sandpit may readily introduce some sand into the vagina by direct contact with the sand or by the hands. Soreness may be associated with masturbation.

Itching due to *threadworms* may cause some vaginitis. The diagnosis is established by a cellophane smear of the anal region followed by microscopy for threadworm ova.

Vaginitis may be due to *thrush*. This should be suspected if the child has oral thrush, or if she is receiving antibiotic treatment by mouth, or if thrush lesions can be seen on the vulva. The diagnosis may be confirmed by microscopy of a vaginal smear.

Vaginitis may be due to *E. coli*, staphylococci, streptococci or gonorrhoea and probably to virus infections such as herpes. The diagnosis may be made on culture. Pus may be milked down to the vulva by a finger in the rectum.

Trichomonas infection is rare before puberty.

Whenever a child has a purulent vaginal discharge or blood in the discharge, the possibility of a *foreign body* must be remembered. This may be demonstrated by x-ray. If necessary the vagina may be inspected by a Kelly cytoscope.

Henderson and Scott (1966) found soiled toilet paper in the vagina of a child with vaginal discharge. In their review they noted that others had found the following foreign bodies in girls with a vaginal discharge: safety-pins, hairpins, folded paper, crayons, twigs, splinters of wood, cherries, paper-clips, beads, bits of toys, pencil erasers, sand, stones, marbles, cotton, shells, nuts, corks and insects.

A rare cause of vaginal discharge is a tumour.

At puberty some leucorrhoea is physiological and results from oestrogen stimulation.

The specialist should examine the girl, carrying out a bimanual pelvic examination with a finger in the rectum. The child may have to be examined under an anaesthetic.

Dysmenorrhoea

This is rare for two or three years after the onset of menstruation, because of the frequency of anovular menstrual cycles. It can be suggested by the mother or older girls, and the commonest cause of dysmenorrhoea in the young adolescent is psychological.

Menorrhagia

The commonest cause of abnormal uterine bleeding in an adolescent is hyperplasia of the endometrium—a self-limiting condition which does not require treatment.

Other important causes of excessive blood loss are anaemia, blood disease and an incomplete abortion.

References

See p. 287.

Delayed puberty in the boy

By delayed puberty I mean the absence of signs of puberty by the age of seventeen.

The following causes of delayed puberty must be considered:

Normal variation
Familial factors
Malnutrition and severe chronic illness
Pituitary disease
Isolated deficiency of gonadotrophins
Gonadal defects
   Cryptorchidism
   Effect of operation
   Mumps
   Klinefelter's syndrome
   Male pseudohermaphroditism
   Male Turner's syndrome

There are considerable *normal variations* in the age of onset of puberty, often familial. Boys of small build are likely to reach puberty later than those of big build. As in the case of the girl, malnutrition or severe illness may delay the onset of puberty. Obesity does not delay the onset of puberty.

Pituitary disease includes in particular the craniopharyngioma and the chromophobe adenoma. There is severe growth failure. Optic atrophy, particularly unilateral, may point to the diagnosis. The X-ray of the skull is an essential investigation. Fröhlich's syndrome is so rare that it can be virtually ignored; in order to make the diagnosis there must be evidence of disease of the hypothalamus, with polyuria, polydipsia and glycosuria, obesity and dwarfism.

Isolated deficiency of gonadotrophins may be associated with anosmia (Kallman's syndrome). It is also found in the Laurence Moon Biedl syndrome of polydactyly, retinitis pigmentosa and dwarfism. It also occurs in association with neurofibromatosis.

Gonadal defects include the undescended testis, testicular atrophy following postpubertal mumps or an operation, and the Klinefelter's syndrome. In the Klinefelter's syndrome the penis is of normal size, but the testes are small and there is gynaecomastia. The diagnosis is confirmed by the buccal smear and chromosome studies.

The male Turner's syndrome is characterised by genital under-development, shortness of stature, webbing of the neck, a low posterior hair line, low set ears, mental subnormality, coarctation of the aorta and cubitus valgus. The diagnosis would be established by the buccal smear and chromosome studies.

The cause of delayed puberty should be sought if there are no signs of puberty by the age of seventeen. Investigations required include the X-ray of the skull, tests of pituitary function, the buccal smear, chromosome studies and estimation of the 17 ketosteroids and urinary gonadotrophins.

References

See p. 287.

Sexual precocity in the girl

Sexual precocity in a girl may be either isosexual or heterosexual. The former implies the early appearance of pubertal features appropriate to the sex of the patient, while the latter implies the development of male secondary sexual characteristics such as enlargement of the clitoris.

The causes of isosexual precocity are as follows:

Constitutional precocious puberty
Intracranial tumours—tumours of the third ventricle, hypothalamic
    tumours; hydrocephalus; hamartoma of the tuber cinereum
Polyostotic fibrous dysplasia
Adrenocortical tumour
Ovarian causes—granulosa cell tumour of the ovary
    Teratomas

Precocious puberty before the age of nine years is the so-called 'constitutional' type, i.e., without any disease, in 90 per cent of cases. It can occur at a few months of age. The sequence of changes may be the same as that of an older child; but the first sign of sexual precocity may be vaginal bleeding alone, pubic hair alone or breast changes, or any combination of these. The child is usually tall for her age at first, but owing to premature closure of the epiphyses, smallness of stature is the end result. It is important that endocrinological investigations should be carried out in order to eliminate the other causes. The investigations include the estimation of the 17 ketosteroids in the urine and urinary gonadotrophins. The 17 ketosteroid output is higher than in ordinary children of the age but normal for puberty. At puberty a vaginal smear shows oestrogenisation.

It should be noted that breast enlargement may occur without other signs of puberty in normal children, and pubic hair can occur without breast enlargement or other signs of puberty. In these cases the stature is average, and the urinary 17 ketosteroids are normal for the age. Gonadotrophins are either not found in the urine or at a low level normal for the age. When there is breast enlargement without any other sign of puberty (premature thelarche) the areola is usually pale and unpigmented.

Sometimes vaginal bleeding without pubic hair may occur in a young child, and not recur for some years until normal adolescence occurs (Seckel, 1960). The stature would be average for the age, and there would be no oestrogenisation in the vaginal smear.

Intracranial conditions should be revealed in the ordinary physical examination of the child, including ophthalmoscopy for papilloedema. Investigations include an x-ray of skull for abnormal calcification and alterations in the sella, EEG, and if necessary an echogram, carotid angiogram or air study.

Polyostotic fibrous dysplasia (Albright's syndrome) consists of precocious puberty, pigmentation of one side of the body (perhaps only a patch on the buttocks or thigh), with x-ray evidence of fibrous dysplasia in the femur or other bones on the same side as the pigmentation. The exact mechanism of the precocious puberty is uncertain. Vaginal bleeding commonly precedes other signs of precocity.

When the cause of precocious puberty is an *ovarian tumour*, the vaginal bleeding tends to be marked, with minimal breast changes and pubic hair. The diagnosis should be suspected if vaginal bleeding precedes the development of pubic hair or of breast changes. The tumour is usually felt on bimanual examination. If there is a granulosa cell tumour, there is a great excess of oestrogens in the urine, and in the case of a teratoma there is an excessive output of gonadotrophins from the tumour.

Heterosexual precocity is due to adrenocortical hyperplasia or tumour.

Adrenocortical tumours usually make themselves obvious by the rapid onset of puberty, often with the full appearance of Cushing's syndrome, obesity of the buffalo type, with little fat in the extremities, a plethoric facies, hypertension, commonly stunting of growth and hypertrichosis. There is an excess of 17 hydroxycorticosteroids in the urine. The common cause is a carcinoma.

Precocious puberty also occurs in association with *adrenocortical hyperplasia*, which is normally associated with pseudohermaphroditism. There is enlargement of the clitoris from birth, usually with advanced skeletal maturation and increased 17 ketosteroids in the urine.

References

See p. 287.

Sexual precocity in the boy

Whereas in 90 per cent of cases of sexual precocity in girls the cause is 'constitutional' and not related to disease, the majority of cases in boys are due to serious disease.

As a rule, if the penis is fully developed as at puberty, and the testes are normal in size for puberty, the cause is likely to be intracranial. If the penis is large but the testes are small and undeveloped, the cause is likely to be in the adrenal.

The causes are:

Intracranial—tumours involving the hypothalamus

Adrenal—hyperplasia or carcinoma

Testicular—teratoma, etc

Hydrocephalus

Postencephalitis

As in the girl, an *intracranial tumour* may be indicated by ophthalmoscopic examination and the same investigations are necessary.

References

ALTCHEK A. (1972) Premature Thelarche. *Pediatric Clinics N. Amer.*, **19,** 543.

DEWHURST C.J. (1963) *Gynaecological disorders of infants and children.* London, Cassell.

FEDERMAN D.D. (1967) *Abnormal Sexual Development.* Philadelphia, Saunders.

FLUHMANN C.F. (1958) Menstrual problems of adolescence. *Pediatric Clinics N. America,* Feb. 1958, p. 51.

HUBBLE D. (1969) *Paediatric Endocrinology.* Oxford, Blackwell Scientific Publications.

JONES H.W., HELLER R.H. (1966) *Pediatric and Adolescent Gynecology.* Baltimore, Williams and Wilkins.

McARTHUR J.W., TRUMAN J.T. & CONNOLLY J.P. (1964) Common menstrual disorders in the adolescent girl. *Clin. Pediatrics,* **3,** 663.

SECKEL H.P.G. (1960) Premature thelarche and premature metrarche followed by normal adolescence. *J. Pediat.,* **57,** 204.

SIGURJONSDOTTIR T.J. & HAYLES A.B. (1968) Precocious Puberty. *Am. J. Dis. Child.,* **115,** 309.

WIDHOLM O. (1965) Menstrual disorders in adolescence. *Clin. Pediatrics,* **5,** 118.

WILKINS L. (1965) *The Diagnosis and Treatment of Endocrine Disorders in Childhood and Adolescence.* Springfield, Charles Thomas.

Gynaecomastia

When a boy has enlargement of the breast, the following conditions have to be considered:

Normal newborn breast enlargement
Normal gynaecomastia of adolescence
Disease involving the skin, pituitary, thyroid, lung, adrenal, liver, kidney, testis. Malnutrition. Paraplegia
Effect of drugs
Klinefelter's syndrome

Enlargement of the breast is normal in newborn full term male babies, but rare in prematurely born ones. An obese boy may appear to have breast enlargement, while in fact the appearance is due to nothing more than fatty tissue.

Gynaecomastia is common in *adolescence*. In a study of 1855 non obese adolescent boys, it was found in 38·7 per cent. The figure for the 14–14½ year old group was 64·6 per cent. In 23·3 per cent the enlargement was unilateral. It persisted for up to 2 years in 27·1 per cent and up to 3 years in 7·7 per cent (Nydick *et al.*, 1961).

Gynaecomastia is occasionally seen in various diseases in adults, including generalised skin conditions, severe malnutrition, acromegaly, thyrotoxicosis, carcinoma of the lung, feminising adrenocortical tumour, cirrhosis of the liver, renal failure, or tumour of the testis. It may occur in paraplegic patients. It is not clear how many of these conditions cause gynaecomastia in children.

The following *drugs* may cause gynaecomastia: amphetamine, anabolic steroids, digitalis, gonadotrophins, imipramine, isoniazid, oestrogens, P.A.S., phenothiazines, progesterone, reserpine, spironolactone, testosterone, vincristine.

Gynaecomastia may be a feature of *Klinefelter's syndrome*. Some 25 per cent of such children are mentally subnormal. The testes are small for the age. The diagnosis is established by the buccal smear and chromosome analysis.

References

STEINER M.M. (1955) Enlargement of breasts during childhood. *Pediat. Clin. N. Am.*, May, p. 575.
NYDICK M., BUSTOS J., DALE J.H. & RAWSON R.W. (1961) Gynecomastia in Adolescent Boys. *J. Am. med. Ass.*, **178**, 449.
Annotation. Gynaecomastia (1964) *Brit. med. J.*, **2**, 1548.

Pruritus

Pruritus, or the itch, is a common symptom in childhood. Perhaps the commonest causes are infantile eczema or urticaria, irritation by contact with wool or a sweat rash. The following are the main causes to consider:

Irritation by wool next to skin
Sweat rash
Urticaria
Insect bites
Pediculosis
Ringworm infection
Chilblains
Threadworms (pruritus ani)
Scabies
Pyogenic skin infections
Chickenpox
Eczema
Psoriasis
Lichen planus
Pityriasis rosea
Dermatitis herpetiformis
Serum sickness
Mycosis fungoides
Jaundice
Uraemia
Leukaemia

Reticuloses
Diabetes mellitus
Psychological factors
Drugs

There are other conditions which cause pruritus, but the above are the principal ones. The list is such a long one that it would not be profitable to discuss the differential diagnosis. Urticaria and the effect of drugs will alone be mentioned further.

The most common cause of urticaria is sensitivity to insect bites, such as the fleas from a dog or cat or other household pet. It may also be due to foods or inhalants, and to a wide variety of drugs.

Innumerable *drugs* may cause urticaria or pruritus. They include amitriptyline, antibiotics, antihistamines, anisera, aspirin, barbiturates, codeine, chloroquine, colistin, dichloralphenazone, diphenoxylate, gold, imipramine, indomethacin, methimazole, nalidixic acid, phenothiazines, phenytoin, quinine, tetanus toxoid, vitamin A and corticosteroid ointment.

Loss of hair

Loss of hair may be due to the following conditions:

Head rolling
Trichotillomania
Alopecia areata
Ringworm and other infections
Thyroid and pituitary deficiency
Abnormalities of hair structure—trichorrhexis, pili torti, monilethrix
Any severe chronic illness

Rare syndromes
   Ectodermal dysplasia
   Progeria
   Dystrophia myotonica
   Argininosuccinicaciduria
   Other rare syndromes

Drugs

Infants often denude their heads in a patch or patches by *head rolling*. Toddlers and other children sometimes acquire the habit of pulling their hair out; it is usually a manifestation of insecurity.

Alopecia areata may be due to several causes. The hair tends to break off 2 to 3 mm from the root. The broken hair is the shape of an exclamation mark, being thicker at the top than the base.

Ringworm is diagnosed by fluorescence under Wood's light or by detection of the fungi in potassium hydroxide on a slide.

Thyroid and pituitary deficiency including the Laurence Moon Biedl syndrome may be associated with hair loss.

Trichorrhexis nodosa is a condition in which there are nodular swellings on the hair with fractures of the hair shaft. *Pili torti* consist of twisted hairs. The condition is hereditary and is sometimes associated with deafness. Affected infants are commonly born without hair. After some growth of hair, the eyelashes, hair of scalp and hair of eyebrows fall out. *Monilethrix* is a developmental anomaly of the hair shaft. The diagnosis is made by microscopy.

Hair loss may be the sequel of any *chronic illness*.

Numerous *rare syndromes* are associated with hair loss. They are listed in the book by Rook, Wilkinson and Ebling (1968).

Drugs which cause hair loss include amphetamine, anticoagulants, antimetabolities, bismuth, carbamazepine, chloroquine, ethionamide, gentamicin, gold, mepacrine, P.A.S., phenytoin, primidone, propylthiouracil, thallium, troxidone, Vitamin A excess. Hair loss may follow several weeks after anticoagulant therapy.

Excessive hair

Hypertrichosis is often racial. It also occurs in the following conditions:

Cushing's syndrome (p. 26)
Drugs
Porphyria
Lipodystrophy
Epidermolysis bullosa

Mucopolysaccharidoses
Addison's disease
Cornelia de Lange syndrome
Dermatomyositis (p. 38)
Degenerative diseases of the nervous system
Adrenocortical hyperplasia

Various *drugs* cause hypertrichosis. They include diazeoxide, corticosteroids, anabolic steroids, phenytoin, streptomycin and corticosteroid ointment.

Epidermolysis bullosa is a congenital disease in which bullae develop mainly at the site of trauma or pressure. Scars may follow the healing process.

There are several types of mucopolysaccharidoses, including Hurler's syndrome (gargoylism) with progressive hepatosplenomegaly, cataract formation, hirsutism and mental deterioration.

The *Cornelia de Lange* syndrome presents with a characteristic facies in which the eyebrows are continuous with each other, there is hirsutism, malformed hands with a proximal thumb and other defects.

References

FORBES A. (1965) Hypertrichosis. *New Engl. J. Med.*, **273**, 602.

ROOK A., WILKINSON D.S. & EBLING F.J.G. (1968) *Textbook of Dermatology*. Oxford, Blackwell Scientific Publications.

Side effects of drugs

Nearly all drugs may have unpleasant side effects, and it was felt that a book concerning the common symptoms of disease would not be complete without a brief account of the side actions of drugs used to treat disease—side effects which are commonly confused with the results of the disease.

At the risk of some oversimplification, one may group the side effects of drugs as follows, according to the tissue predominantly involved:

(1) Action on the skin—rashes; erythematous, urticarial, scarlatiniform, morbilliform, erythema multiforme, erythema nodosum, exfoliative dermatitis, purpura, acne, striae, photosensitivity, pigmentation, hair loss or hypertrichosis, Stevens Johnson syndrome, disseminated lupus, fixed drug eruptions.

(2) Action on the brain, psychological or otherwise. Advantageous —the patient thinking that he is better, although the drug had no relevant pharmacological action. Disadvantageous— the patient imagining that the drug is causing untoward symptoms. Direct action on the brain—causing confusion or other symptoms.

(3) Action on the eye—causing cataract, optic atrophy, papilloedema, retinal changes, conjuctivitis.

(4) Action on the ear—causing deafness or ataxia.

(5) Action on the heart.

(6) Action on the liver—hepatitis.

(7) Action on the kidney—albuminuria, haematuria, nephrotic syndrome.

(8) Action on the blood.
Predominantly red cells—haemolysis, megaloblastic anaemia, hypoplastic anaemia.
Predominantly white cells—granulopenia, agranulocytosis.

Predominantly platelets—thrombocytopenic purpura.
Action on several of the blood elements.
Action on clotting mechanism.
Action on the haemoglobin—methaemoglobinaemia.

(9) Action on the alimentary tract—abdominal pain, ulceration, bleeding, vomiting, diarrhoea, constipation.
(10) Allergic and anaphylactoid reactions. Asthma.
(11) Drug fever.
(12) Collagen disease—disseminated lupus, periarteritis.
(13) Superinfection—especially moniliasis.
(14) Drug resistance and antagonism.
(15) Drug dependence and addiction.
(16) Action on the foetus when drug taken in pregnancy.

Drug reactions are usually due to overdosage, intolerance, side effects, including secondary effects, idiosyncrasy, hypersensitivity and allergy.

In the section to follow, I have made no attempt to list side effects in order of frequency. This clearly would be impossible. Some of the side effects mentioned are probably rare, but it was felt that a fairly comprehensive list would be useful for the family doctor.

Some rashes caused by drugs

Acne may be caused by bromides, iodides, corticosteroids, phenytoin.

Bullous eruptions may be caused by acetazolamide, barbiturates, bromides, chloral, meprobamate, nalidixic acid, phenytoin, salicylates, sulphonamides, thiazide diuretics, tricyclic antidepressants (e.g., imipramine).

Erythema nodosum may be caused by penicillin, salicylates, sulphonamides and thiouracil, and develop when corticosteroids are withdrawn.

Exfoliative dermatitis may be caused by anticonvulsants, barbiturates, chloroquine, gold, griseofulvin, penicillin, phenothiazines, salicylates, sulphonamides, thiouracil.

Fixed drug eruptions may be caused by anticonvulsants, antihistamines, barbiturates, iodides, penicillin, salicylates, sulphonamides, tetracycline.

Photosensitivity rashes may be caused by antidepressants, antiemetic drugs, antihistamines, barbiturates, cytotoxic drugs, diphenhydramine, nalidixic acid, phenothiazines, sulphonamides, tetracycline, thiazide diuretics.

Pigmentation may be caused by antimalarial drugs, corticosteroids, cytotoxic drugs, gold, mercury, phenothiazines, phenytoin, vitamin A excess.

Toxic epidermal necrolysis may be due to barbiturates, nitrofurantoin, penicillin, phenytoin, sulphonamides.

Side effects of individual drugs

(Some of the side effects listed are rare. Selected important side effects are in italics)

Acetaminophen (Paracetamol)—granulopenia, hypoglycaemia.

Acetazolamide (Diamox)—action on blood, kidney, liver; confusion, depression, diarrhoea, drowsiness, excitement, fever, fits, glycosuria, haematuria, headaches, irritability, melaena, paraesthesiae, polydipsia, rash, renal calculus, vertigo, vomiting.

Actinomycin D—*action on blood, alopecia,* diarrhoea, intestinal ulceration, oral ulcers, rash.

Adrenaline—*fainting, nervousness, pallor, sweating,* tremor.

Aminophylline—*agitation,* anxiety, coma, *death,* dehydration, delirium, fever, fits, haematemesis, haematuria, headache, overventilation, rashes, respiratory paralysis, restlessness, shock, thirst, vomiting.

Amitriptyline (Tryptizol)—abdominal pain, action on blood and liver; ataxia, blurring of vision, constipation, drowsiness, dry mouth, excitement, fatigue, fever, fits, headache, mouth ulcers, nausea, numbness, oedema of face, oliguria, paraesthesiae, pruritus, rash, sweating, tremors, vertigo, vomiting, weakness.

Amphetamine—aggressiveness, *anorexia,* drowsiness, *drug dependence,* dry mouth, hyperthermia, *insomnia,* irritability, jaundice, paranoia, pupils dilated, rash, sweating, tremor.

Ampicillin (Penbritin)—see Penicillin.

Anabolic steroids, e.g., Methandienone (Dianabol), Norethandrolone (Nilevar)—*jaundice,* lowered P.B.I., *premature closure of epiphyses,* raised serum lipoids.

Anthisan—see Antihistamines.

Antihistamines—action on blood, amblyopia, confusion, *drowsiness, dry mouth,* dysuria, fainting, fits, frequency of micturition, gastric disturbance, hallucinations, headache, insomnia, irritability, tachycardia, urinary retention, vertigo.

Aspirin—see Salicylates.

Atebrin—see Mepacrine.

Azathioprine (Imuran)—abdominal pain, *action on blood* and liver; fever, herpes, nausea, rash, pancreatitis, vomiting.

Bacitracin—action on kidney, anorexia, nausea, pain at site of injection, rash.

Barbiturates—amblyopia, *bad behaviour* (especially in mentally subnormal child), *concentration impaired, drowsiness, drug dependence,* hepatosplenomegaly, *insomnia, irritability,* megaloblastic anaemia, nystagmus, purpura, *rash,* Stevens Johnson syndrome; withdrawal symptoms—delirium, fits, tremors.

Bephenium—diarrhoea, nausea, vomiting.

Betamethazone—see Corticosteroids.

Boric acid—death, diarrhoea and vomiting, haemorrhages, peripheral circulatory failure, red beefy rash.

Calcium chloride—*gastric irritation.*

Capreomycin—action on kidney, deafness, defective colour vision, hypocalcaemia, hypokalaemia, optic neuritis.

Carbamazepine (Tegretol)—*action on blood,* amblyopia, diarrhoea, diplopia, disseminated lupus, dizziness, drowsiness, fits, purpura, rash, Stevens Johnson syndrome, vomiting.

Carbenicillin—see Penicillin.

Cephalosporins—abdominal discomfort, action on blood, kidney and liver; allergy, anorexia, diarrhoea, fever, nausea, oedema, Parkinsonism, rash, serum sickness like symptoms, superinfection, thrombophlebitis at injection site, vomiting, wheezing.

Ceporin—see Cephalosporins.

Chlorambucil—cataract.

Chloramphenicol—newborn baby—abdominal distension, cyanosis, death, flaccidity, *grey syndrome*—failure to thrive, hypothermia, irregular respirations, loose stools, pruritus, vomiting.

Other children—*action on the blood*, especially granulopenia; action on liver; optic neuritis, peripheral neuritis.

Chlordiazepoxide (Librium)—abdominal discomfort, action on blood and liver; anorexia, ataxia, constipation, drowsiness, *extrapyramidal symptoms*, hypotension, mania, memory impaired, nausea, oedema, overactivity, rashes, urinary difficulty, vertigo, vomiting.

Chloromycetin—see Chloramphenicol.

Chloroquine—accommodation impaired, action on blood and liver; *blurred vision*, burning in epigastrium, burning in mouth, *cataract*, hair loss and loss of colour, myopathy, nausea, rashes, *retinal changes* (maybe delayed for 4–5 years), vomiting.

Chlorothiazide group—action on blood, allergy, cramp, hyperglycaemia, melaena, pancreatitis, *potassium loss*, vertigo.

Chlorpheniramine (Piriton)—see Antihistamines.

Chlorpromazine (Largactil)—see Phenothiazines.

Cloxacillin—see Penicillin.

Codeine—collapse of lung if cough productive, drying of secretions.

Colistin—*action on kidney, deafness*, muscle weakness, nystagmus, paraesthesiae, vertigo.

Corticosteroids—*acne*, agranulocytosis, *cataract, Cushing's syndrome, death sudden*, delayed healing, *dermal atrophy, diabetes*, fits, glaucoma, *growth inhibition, hypertension, increased severity of chickenpox, muscle weakness, obesity, operative shock, osteoporosis*, pancreatitis, panniculitis, *peptic ulcer, purpura, sodium retention, striae, suppression of pain in infection*, thrombocytopenia, thromboembolic phenomena.

On discontinuing—increased intracranial pressure.

Skin applications—*acne*, burning sensation, *dermal atrophy*, folliculitis, hypertrichosis, miliaria, pruritus, *striae*.

Cortisone—see Corticosteroids.

Corticotrophin (ACTH)—same as corticosteroids; more tendency to acne, allergy, hirsutism, hypertension, pigmentation: less bruising, less dyspepsia, osteoporosis, striae.

Cotrimoxazole—see trimethoprim.

Cyclopentolate—*acute psychosis*, ataxia, delirium, dry mouth, visual hallucinations.

Cyclophosphamide—*action on blood* and liver; *alopecia*, amenorrhoea, anorexia, *cystitis*, *diarrhoea*, headache, intestinal ulceration, malignant disease, myelitis, nausea, oral ulcers, pneumonitis, protein losing enteropathy, pulmonary fibrosis, *sterility*, vomiting.

Cycloserine—action on blood, fits, neurotoxic, psychoses.

Demethylchlortetracycline (Ledermycin)—facial oedema, *photosensitivity, staining of teeth*.

Dexamethasone—see Corticosteroids.

Diamox—see Acetazolamide.

Diazepam (Valium)—action on blood and liver; acute excitement, ataxia, depression, diplopia, drowsiness, dysarthria, hallucinations, headache, nausea, rash, *respiratory depression*, temperature fall, tremors, vertigo.

Diazoxide—*hypertrichosis*.

Dichloralphenazone—pruritus.

Dichlorophen—abdominal discomfort, diarrhoea, rash, urticaria, vomiting.

Digoxin—*bradycardia, coupling of the beats*, nausea, *oliguria*, scotoma, *vomiting*, xanthopsia.

Diphenoxylate (Lomotil)—ataxia, depression, dizziness, drowsiness, insomnia, nausea, nystagmus, pruritus, rash, vomiting

Dulcolax—see oxphenisatin.

Epanutin—see Phenytoin.

Ephedrine—headache, *insomnia*, nausea, *nervousness*, pallor, palpitation, sweating, tremor.

Equanil—see Meprobamate.

Ergotamine—chilling of extremities, *gangrene*, headache, nausea, *numbness, tingling*, vomiting.

Erythromycin—abdominal pain, allergy, diarrhoea, *jaundice* (mainly the estolate), nausea, rash, vomiting, wheezing.

Ethacrynic acid—electrolyte disturbance, pancreatitis, ventricular fibrillation.

Ethambutol—gastrointestinal symptoms, loss of colour vision, rash, reduced visual activity, retrobulbar neuritis.

Ethamivan (Vandid)—*convulsions*.

Ethionamide—abdominal pain, acne, alopecia, anorexia, diarrhoea, jaundice, mental changes, peripheral neuritis, photosensitivity, salivation, vomiting.

Ethosuccimide (Zarontin)—abdominal pain, action on blood, kidney and liver; anorexia, depression, disseminated lupus, drowsiness, fatigue, headache, hiccough, nausea, psychosis, rash, stomatitis, vaginal bleeding, vomiting.

Fenfluramine—confusion, diarrhoea, drowsiness, dyskinesis, lethargy, nightmares, poor concentration, toothgrinding; withdrawal—*agitation*.

Flufenamic acid—diarrhoea.

Framycetin—deafness.

Fucidin—see Sodium fusidate.

Furadantin—see Nitrofurantoin.

Gentamicin—*action on ears, kidney*, alopecia, blurred vision, permanent vestibular damage.

Gold—*action on blood, kidney, liver*; pruritus, *rashes*, stomatitis.

Griseofulvin—action on blood, kidney, liver, stomach; disseminated lupus, headache, insomnia, peripheral neuritis, photosensitivity, poor concentration, superinfection, vertigo.

Hyoscine—*atropine like action*, coma, dryness of mouth, excitement, hallucination.

Ibuprofen—dyspepsia.

Imipramine (Tofranil)—abdominal pain, accommodation impaired, action on blood and liver, anxiety, cold extremities, concentration impaired, constipation, delirium, difficulty in micturition, drowsiness, dryness of mucous membranes, dysarthria, dysphagia, fits, giddiness, glossitis, gynaecomastia, insomnia, irritability, nausea, oliguria, palpitation, Parkinsonism, postural hypotension, pruritus, pulmonary infiltration, rashes, sudden falls, sweating, tachycardia, tearfulness, tremors, vertigo.

Imuran—see Azathioprine.

Indocid—see Indomethacin.

Indomethacin (Indocid)—action on blood and liver, anorexia, asthma, ataxia, blurred vision, buccal ulcer, confusion, corneal and retinal changes, death, drowsiness, diarrhoea, headache, nausea, oedema, pancreatitis, peptic ulcer, pruritus, psychological changes, rash, vertigo, vomiting.

Iodides—*acne, coryza*, gastric disturbances, goitre, oedema of eye-lids, swelling of salivary glands.

Iron—abdominal discomfort, blackening of teeth and stools, constipation, diarrhoea.

Iron dextran—lymphadenopathy.

Isoniazid—action on blood, kidney, liver; albuminuria, cramp, disseminated lupus, excitability, fits, gynaecomastia, optic atrophy, pancreatitis, *peripheral neuritis*, psychological changes, rash, vertigo, vomiting.

Kanamycin,—action on blood, ear, kidney, liver; amblyopia, diarrhoea, paraesthesiae, rash, superinfection, tinnitus, vertigo.

Largactil—see Chlorpromazine.

Ledermycin—see Demethylchlortetracycline.

Librium—see Chlordiazepoxide.

Lincomycin—abdominal pain, action on blood and liver; diarrhoea, muscle pain, overgrowth of yeasts, pruritus, rashes, superinfection, vomiting.

Lomotil—see Diphenoxylate.

Mefenamic acid—diarrhoea, dyspepsia, haemolysis, leucopenia, rash.

Mellaril (Thioridazine)—see Phenothiazines.

Mepacrine (Atebrin) action on blood, psychosis, *yellow staining of skin.*

Meprobamate (Miltown, equanil)—action on blood, agitation, anaphylactoid reaction, anorexia, ataxia, blurred vision, bronchospasm, depression, drowsiness, drug dependence, fever, frequency, gastroenteritis, lymphadenopathy, Parkinsonism, proctitis, rash, stomatitis, thirst, vertigo, vomiting. Withdrawal—insomnia, tremors, twitching.

Mepyramine (Anthisan)—see Antihistamines.

6-Mercaptopurine—action on blood, liver; anorexia, diarrhoea, intestinal ulceration, oral ulcers, vomiting.

Methimazole—action on blood and liver; arthralgia, C.N.S. depression or stimulation, fever, hypothyroidism, oedema, pruritus, rash

Methotrexate—abdominal pain, action on blood and liver; alopecia, diarrhoea, lung infiltration, melaena, nausea, oral ulceration, rash, renal tubular damage, vomiting.

Methylphenidate (Ritalin)—anxiety, dyspepsia, headache, palpitation, rash, tremors.

Milontin—see Phensuccimide.

Miltown—see Meprobamate.

Mogadon—see Nitrazepam.

Morphia—nausea, vomiting.

Mysoline—see Primidone.

Nalidixic acid (Negram)—anaemia, diarrhoea, drowsiness, false positive for urinary reducing substances, fits, glycosuria, haemolysis, headache, hyperglycaemia, hypertension, increased intracranial pressure, jaundice, muscle weakness, myalgia, nausea, paraesthesiae, photosensitivity, polyarthritis, pruritus, rash, sixth nerve weakness and squint, vertigo, visual disturbance, vomiting.

Negram—see Nalidixic acid.

Neomycin—action on ear, kidney, and liver; steatorrhoea, wheezing.

Nitrazepam (Mogadon)—ataxia, bronchial hypersecretion, drowsiness, increased appetite, lachrymation, salivation.

Nitrofurantoin—action on blood, kidney and liver; alopecia, anaphylaxis, angioneurotic oedema, chills, eosinophilia, fever, haemolysis in presence of glucose 6 phosphate dehydrogenase deficiency, hallucinations, headache, muscle pains, nausea, paraesthesiae, peripheral neuritis, pleural effusion, pulmonary infiltration, rash, teeth discoloured, vomiting.

Nortriptyline—action similar to amitriptyline. Also deafness.

Novobiocin—action on blood and liver; rash, yellow staining of skin.

Nystatin—abdominal pain, diarrhoea.

Oleandomycin—jaundice.

Ospolot—see Sulthiame.

Oxyphenisation (Dulcolax)—lupoid hepatitis.

P.A.S. (Para-amino salicylic acid)—abdominal pain, action on blood, kidney and liver; diarrhoea, disseminated lupus, drowsiness, fever, gynaecomastia, haemorrhages, hair loss, lymphadenopathy, optic atrophy, photophobia, pulmonary infiltration, rash, steatorrhoea, thyroid enlargement, vitamin B deficiency, vomiting.

Paracetamol—granulopenia.

Paromomycin—abdominal pain, action on kidney, deafness, diarrhoea, headache, nausea, rash, steatorrhoea, superinfection, vertigo, vomiting.

Penbritin—see Ampicillin.

Penicillin—*anaphylaxis*, angioneurotic oedema, arthralgia, asthma, conjunctivitis, *diarrhoea* when taken by mouth, effusion into joints, *haemolysis*, increased intracranial pressure, lachrymation, limb pain, periarteritis, polyneuritis, pruritus, rashes, superinfection, wheezing.

Perphenazine (Fentazin)—see Phenothiazine.

Pethidine—nausea, vertigo.

Phenacetin—jaundice.

Pheneturide—action on blood, kidney and liver; ataxia, dyspepsia, rash.

Phenobarbitone—see Barbiturates.

Phenothiazine group of tranquillisers (Chlorpromazine (Largactil), Perphenazine (Fentazin), Promazine (Sparine), Thioridazine (Melleril), Trifluoperazine (Stelazine))—action on blood and liver; catatonia, concentration impaired, constipation, *corneal opacities,* constriction of chest, diarrhoea, drowsiness, *extrapyramidal symptoms*, fever, fits, gynaecomastia, headache, lactorrhoea, muscle rigidity, neck stiffness, oculogyric crises, opisthotonos, postural hypotension, paralysis of accommodation, photosensitivity, pigmentation of retina and skin, pruritus, rash, rigidity, stomatitis, sweating, tremors, vertigo.

Phensuccimide (Milontin)—action on blood, ataxia, disseminated lupus erythematosus, drowsiness, haematuria, hepatosplenomegaly, lymphadenopathy, nausea, rash, vertigo.

Phenylazopyridine (pyridium)—action on blood, yellow urine.

Phenylbutazone—action on blood, lymphadenopathy.

Phenytoin (Epanutin)—abdominal discomfort, action on blood, kidney and liver; alopecia, amblyopia, anorexia, arthropathy, *ataxia*, conjunctivitis, constipation, decalcification, diplopia, disseminated lupus, drowsiness, dysarthria, *gingivitis*, haematuria, hair loss, headache, hepatosplenomegaly, *hirsutism*, hyperglycaemia, interaction with phenobarbitone, phenothiazines, P.A.S., sulthiame; joint effusion, lymphadenopathy, lymphoma, megaloblastic anaemia, mental slowing, nausea, *nystagmus*, periarteritis, pigmentation, pruritus, rash, rickets, skull thickening, Stevens Johnson syndrome, striae, tremors, vomiting.

Piperazine—abdominal pain, accommodation impaired, allergic purpura, ataxia, blurring of vision, coma, confusion, hallucination, hypotonia, incoordination, muscle weakness, paraesthesiae, precipitation of fits in epileptics, rashes, tremors, vertigo, vomiting.

Piriton—see Chlorpheniramine.

Polymyxin—action on kidney, ataxia, circumoral numbness, fever, neurotoxic, paraesthesiae, pruritus, rash, slurred speech, vertigo.

Ponderax—see Fenfluramine.

Prednisone—see Corticosteroids.

Primidone (Mysoline)—abdominal pain, action on blood, alopecia, amblyopia, angioneurotic oedema, ataxia, decalcification, diplopia, disseminated lupus, *drowsiness*, dysarthria, hair loss, *irritability*, lymphadenopathy, megaloblastic, anaemia, nausea, *nystagmus*, oedema of eyelids, overactivity, psychoses, rash, vertigo, vomiting.

Promazine (Sparine)—see Phenothiazine.

Pyopen (Carbenicillin)—see Penicillin.

Pyrazinamide—action on liver, limb pains.

Pyridium—see Phenylazopyridine.

Quinine—deafness, jaundice, tinnitus.

Rifampicin—abdominal pain, action on blood and liver; bone pain, diarrhoea, drowsiness, dyspepsia, dyspnoea, fever, headache, nausea, rash; red urine, sputum, tears; vomiting, wheezing.

Ristocetin—action on blood and kidney, albuminuria, thromboses.

Ritalin—see Methylphenidate.

Salbutamol—tremors.

Salicylates—*anaemia, angioneurotic oedema, asthma*, bleeding by causing hypoprothrombinaemia or thrombocytopenia, deafness, haematemesis, increase of chronic urticaria, jaundice, nystagmus, *overventilation, tinnitus*, vertigo, vomiting. Aspirin particles also cause bleeding by direct action on gastric mucosa.

Sodium fusidate—diarrhoea, vomiting.

Sparine (Promazine)—see Phenothiazine.

Stelazine (Trifluoperazine)—see Phenothiazine.

Streptomycin—*ataxia, deafness*, fever, muscle weakness, paraesthesiae, pruritus, rash, wheezing.

Sulphasalazine—action on blood, anorexia, fever, headache, muscle pain, nausea, rash, vomiting.

Sulphonamides—*action on blood and liver*; *crystalluria*, disseminated lupus, *drug fever*, headache, lymphadenopathy, myopia, nausea, necrotising angiitis, optic neuritis, pancreatitis, photosensitivity, polyarteritis, polyneuritis, pulmonary infiltration, rash, vertigo.

   Long acting sulphonamides—*Stevens Johnson syndrome.*

Sulthiame (Ospolot)—action on blood and kidney; anorexia, ataxia, blurred vision, confusion, drowsiness, dysarthria, headache, loss of weight, *overventilation*, paraesthesiae, photophobia, psychotic excitement, renal calculus, status epilepticus, vertigo.

Synacthen—see Corticotrophin.

Tegretol—see Carbamazepine.

Testosterone group—acne, jaundice, premature closure of epiphyses, virilisation.

Tetanus Toxoid—dysarthria, erythema around smallpox scar, peripheral neuritis, pruritus, sweating, urticaria, wheezing.

Tetracyclines—abdominal pain, anaphylaxis, *bulging fontanelle*, *diarrhoea*, disseminated lupus, *enamel hypoplasia*, enterocolitis, fever, glossitis, jaundice, myopia, *overgrowth of monilia*, pancreatitis, peptic ulcer, *photosensitivity*, pruritus, rash, *tooth and nail discolouration*, wheezing.

   Old stocks—abnormal aminoaciduria, Fanconi-like syndrome, nausea, oedema, polydipsia, polyuria, vomiting.

Thiobendazole—dyspepsia, headache, hyperglycaemia, leucopenia, numbness, pruritus, tinnitus, vertigo, xanthopsia.

Thioridazine (Melleril)—see Phenothiazines.

Thiouracil—acne, action on blood and liver; disseminated lupus, fever, lymphadenopathy, rash.

Thyroxin—*heart failure at onset, loss of weight.*

   Overdose—*advanced skeletal maturation followed by premature closure of epiphyses, diarrhoea, irritability, tachycardia.*

Tofranil—see Imipramine.

Tranquillisers and antidepressants—see chlordiazepoxide, chlorpromazine, imipramine, meprobamate, methylphenidate, phenothiazine group.

Triamcinolone—see Costicosteroids.

Tridione—see Troxidone.

Trifluoperazine (Stelazine)—see Phenothiazines.

Trimeprazine (Vallergan)—abdominal pain, depression, drowsiness, dry mouth, headache, nasal stuffiness, rash, vertigo.

Trimethoprim—action on blood, diarrhoea, headache, nausea, paraesthesiae, vertigo, vomiting.

Troxidone—abdominal pain, acne, *action on blood and liver*; alopecia, angioneurotic oedema, diplopia, disseminated lupus, drowsiness, effusion into joints, grand mal, haematuria, headache, hiccoughs, irritability, lymphadenopathy, *nephrotic syndrome*, photophobia, rash, Stevens Johnson syndrome, vomiting, white vision.

Tryptizol—see Amitriptyline.

Valium—see Diazepam.

Vancomycin—action on blood, ears, kidney and liver; fever, paraesthesiae, phlebitis, rash, respiratory arrest, rigor, superinfection, thromboses, urticaria.

Vandid—see Ethamivan.

Vincristine—abdominal pain, *action on blood, alopecia*, ataxia, constipation, diarrhoea, headache, hoarseness, insomnia, jaw pain, oral ulcers, pain in fingers, paraesthesiae, peripheral neuritis, pigmentation, ptosis, rash, vomiting.

Viomycin—action on ears, kidney and liver; electrolyte disturbances, rashes.

Viprynium—abdominal pain, diarrhoea, nausea, red stools, vomiting.

Vitamin A excess—abdominal pain, anorexia, arthralgia, *bone pain*, brittle nails, dry mouth, dry skin, fractures, *hepatosplenomegaly*, hydrocephalus, hypoplastic anaemia, increased intracranial pressure, myalgia, oedema of occiput, *periostitis*, pruritus, sparse hair, *stomatitis*, vomiting.

Vitamin D excess—anorexia, *hypercalcaemia*, nephrocalcinosis, polyuria.

Vitamin K excess—*haemolysis, kernicterus*.

Zarontin—see Ethosuccimide.

Psychological and organic

Psychological factors are so commonly associated with organic disease that it is essential to eliminate organic disease before concluding that the cause is entirely psychological. In fact one should never conclude that a symptom is entirely psychological without positive evidence of a psychological disorder and without eliminating organic disease. It is then necessary to see the child again in order to make sure that one is right about the absence of organic disease. The difficulty is that organic disease may cause psychological disorders, and psychological disorders may cause somatic symptoms.

Many psychological symptoms are caused by disease. For instance, infections and other diseases which result in a child necessarily or unnecessarily missing school may lead to the child worrying about dropping behind others in his class—and may even make it difficult for him to return to school. A common example of this is asthma: many parents keep their asthmatic child away from school when he has the slightest wheeze (or even a cold which might perhaps lead to a wheeze), and as a result the child drops behind in his work, worries and wheezes all the more, and so is kept away longer still. It is a difficult vicious circle which must be broken. If a mother is over anxious about the child's health, she makes him neurotic and hypochondriacal.

Many school difficulties which have an organic basis lead to psychological symptoms. Learning disorders commonly present as a behaviour problem such as truancy. Clumsiness of movement commonly leads to unhappiness at school because of the unkindness of teachers who ascribe the child's bad writing to carelessness and naughtiness. Defects of hearing or seeing lead to troublesome behaviour problems because the child is unable to follow the work of the class. A child who finds the work too much for him, either because of a learning difficulty in a particular subject or because his

IQ is lower than that of others in his form or for other reasons, may lose heart, become worried, depressed and insecure.

Epilepsy leads to behaviour difficulties in several ways. The child may be rejected from entry to a school because of the epilepsy, or he may be treated differently from others, being prevented, for example, from swimming. If he suffers from frequent attacks of *petit mal* he may so frequently miss what is being said that he drops behind in his class work. He may have temporal lobe epilepsy, which causes bad behaviour, leading, for instance, to outbursts of temper. It is particularly important to remember that drugs given for epilepsy may make him clumsy, drowsy and irritable and cause poor concentration. Phenobarbitone is particularly liable to cause undue irritability and bad behaviour in certain children.

Overactivity, which is sometimes related to prematurity, events during pregnancy or anoxia at birth, leads to difficulties at school, poor concentration and punishment.

I have had children referred to me for behaviour problems which were due to an intracranial neoplasm or tuberculous meningitis. I have found that some children referred for difficult behaviour were suffering from early chorea.

On p. 1 it is noted that certain diseases which lead to poor physical growth lead to food refusal because of food forcing. For instance, congenital heart disease is commonly associated with defective physical growth. This leads to the mother worrying about the child's small size, and so she tries to make him eat more—and he refuses.

A baby was referred to me on account of excessive crying. He was found to have phenylketonuria, and when the serum phenylalanine was reduced by an appropriate diet his behaviour promptly improved.

Some bad behaviour is due to hypoglycaemia. It is well known that some children (and adults) become bad tempered when hungry. Others behave badly because they are tired as a result of an infection or anaemia.

Chronic diarrhoea, such as occurs in ulcerative colitis, leads to bad temper and irritability. This may lead some to ascribe the ulcerative colitis to a behaviour problem. Admittedly there are often psychological factors in the aetiology of ulcerative colitis.

Several studies have shown that there is a higher incidence of physical handicap in juvenile delinquents than in the normal population. It is now known that the XYY chromosome anomaly may be associated with tallness of stature and delinquency.

Other conditions which may present as behaviour problems include thyrotoxicosis, migraine, anorectal stenosis, bladder neck obstruction, and (rarely) phaeochromocytoma or neuroblastoma.

Children may be embarrassed and unhappy because of their ugliness or other aspects of their physical appearance, such as obesity, precocious puberty, delayed puberty, short stature or lipodystrophy.

In the next few years we may well learn that more aspects of behaviour have a biochemical or chromosomal basis.

More than half of all the symptoms discussed in this book, all of which may be due to organic disease, may also be psychological in origin. For instance, one of the three components of asthma is psychological disturbance (the other two being allergy and infection). There may be a psychological component in allergic rhinitis. A cough may be merely a habit or an attention seeking device.

Numerous somatic symptoms may arise from psychological problems. They include diarrhoea, abdominal pain, vomiting, frequency of micturition, dysuria, dysmenorrhoea, bed-wetting, polydipsia, polyuria, a poor appetite, indigestion and peptic ulcer, obesity, dirt eating, headache and limb or chest pains. There is a psychological component to several skin conditions, such as eczema, urticaria, lichen planus and pruritus in general. Many other somatic symptoms can be caused by psychological problems.

It has been suggested that psychological factors may influence the resistance to infectious disease (Friedman & Glasgow, 1966).

Reference

FRIEDMAN S.B. & GLASGOW L.A. (1966) Psychologic factors and resistance to infectious disease. *Pediatric Clinics N. America*, 13, 315.

Some symptoms of importance

At the risk of repetition, I propose in this section to enumerate some symptoms of special importance in children, because failure to take note of them may have disastrous results.

Jaundice on the first day, because it requires urgent treatment: it is due to haemolytic disease until proved otherwise. Severe jaundice in the newborn period calls for urgent investigation.

Vomitus containing bile in the newborn period, or vomiting with abdominal distension, suggests intestinal obstruction.

Blood in a baby's vomitus suggests hiatus hernia or reflux, and calls for investigation.

Diarrhoea in any infant or young child is important because of the rapidity with which dehydration may occur.

Stridor of acute onset is important because of the rapidity with which it may get worse and cause complete obstruction.

Cough of really sudden onset, without an upper respiratory infection, suggests an inhaled foreign body.

Ear pain, due to otitis media, requires immediate antibiotic treatment (and *not* drops in the ear).

Neck stiffness (in flexion) suggests meningitis. It is essential to have a lumbar puncture carried out before any antibiotic is given, so that if it is due to pyogenic meningitis the organism can be isolated and the appropriate treatment can be given.

Fits with fever are important because although febrile convulsions are the most likely diagnosis, they may be due to pyogenic meningitis. Hence a lumbar puncture must be performed.

The onset of drowsiness with an infection may represent pyogenic meningitis.

Loss of weight is important because of the many serious causes which could be responsible.

A severe attack of asthma, not responding to the usual treatment.

Poisoning of any kind is important because hospital investigation
and treatment are needed. The dangerous latent period, between the time of ingestion of the poison and the onset of
symptoms, is a particular hazard. Unexplained abnormal
excitement, drowsiness, convulsions or vomiting should be
regarded as due to an overdose of drugs or poisoning until
proved otherwise.

Some popular fallacies

In this section are listed some common errors made when diagnosing
the cause of some of the symptoms mentioned in this book.

Vomiting, crying, green stools or diarrhoea are *not* due to breast
milk not suiting the baby. The only exceptions to this are the
exceedingly rare conditions galactosaemia or lactose intolerance.
If these are suspected the child should be referred to a paediatrician
for the appropriate tests. Green stools in fully breast fed babies do
not suggest an abnormality.

Vomiting, crying, or diarrhoea are *not* due to the breast milk being
too strong for the baby—or not strong enough.

Vomiting, crying or diarrhoea in a full term breast fed or bottle fed
baby are *not* due to overfeeding.

Vomiting, crying or diarrhoea are *not* due to the particular dried
food or other properly constituted feed not suiting the baby.
Nothing will be achieved by changing from one dried food to
another. The child may, however, be intolerant of certain carbohydrates. The child with coeliac disease is probably intolerant of
gluten. The child with hypercalcaemia is intolerant of ordinary
foods and requires a special low calcium milk. A very occasional
baby is sensitive to milk protein.

Infrequent stools in a well breast fed baby are *not* due to constipation. They are normal.

True constipation in an artificially fed baby is *not* due to insufficiency of roughage in the diet. It may be due to inadequate

fluid, inadequate sugar (when the baby is having nothing but milk) or to other factors.

Crying at night in the older baby is *not* due to indigestion or wind. It is almost certainly due to mismanagement and habit formation.

A poor appetite in a well child is almost certainly *not* due to disease —though routine physical and urine examination should be carried out; it is almost certainly due to food forcing.

Bed wetting after the age of three, when it has always occurred, is almost certainly *not* merely psychological in origin, or due to jealousy or faulty management—though psychological problems can readily be added to the basic problem of delayed maturation.

Constant dribbling incontinence is *not* due to delayed maturation; in the boy it is usually due to urethral valves, and in the girl to an ectopic ureter in the vagina, or a ureterocele.

Teething does *not* cause bronchitis, convulsions, fever or diarrhoea.

Delayed walking is *not* a problem for the orthopaedic specialist. It is *not* due to congenital dislocation of the hip.

Delayed talking is *not* due to tongue-tie, laziness, 'everything being done for him', and almost certainly not due to jealousy. If the child is mentally normal, it is usually a familial feature, but may be due to deafness.

Obesity is almost certainly *not* due to the excessively rare condition of Fröhlich's syndrome. I have not yet seen a case.

Some relevant books

APLEY J. (1959) *The Child with Abdominal Pain*. Oxford, Blackwell Scientific Publications.

BAKWIN H., BAKWIN R.M. (1966) *Clinical Management of Behavior Disorders in Children*. Philadelphia, Saunders.

BLACK J.A. (1972) *Neonatal Emergencies and other Problems*. London, Butterworth.

FORD F.R. (1966) *Diseases of the Nervous System in Infancy, Childhood and Adolescence*. Springfield, Charles C. Thomas.

ILLINGWORTH R.S. (1972) *The Normal Child*, Fifth Edition. London, Churchill Livingstone.

ILLINGWORTH R.S. (1964) *The Normal School Child. His Problems Physical and Emotional*. London, Heinemann.

ILLINGWORTH R.S. (1972) *Development of the Infant and Young Child, Normal and Abnormal*. Fifth Edition. London, Churchill Livingstone.

JONES P.G. (1970) *Clinical Paediatric Surgery*. Bristol, Wright.

LAGOS J.C. (1971) *Differential Diagnosis in Paediatric Neurology*. Boston, Little, Brown and Co.

MEYLER L. (1966) *Side Effects of Drugs*. Amsterdam, Excerpta Medica Foundation.

NELSON W.E., VAUGHAN V.C. & McKAY R.J. (1969) *Textbook of Pediatrics*. Philadelphia, Saunders.

ROOK A., WILKINSON D.S. & EBLING F.J.G. (1968) *Textbook of Dermatology*. Oxford, Blackwell Scientific Publications.

SCHAFFER A.J. & AVERY M.E. (1971) *Diseases of the Newborn*. Philadelphia, Saunders.

SCOTT BROWN W.G., BALLANTYNE J., GROVES J. (1965) *Diseases of the Ear, Nose and Throat*. London, Butterworths.

SHERLOCK S. (1968) *Diseases of the Liver and Biliary System*. Fourth Edition. Oxford, Blackwell Scientific Publications.

WADE O.L. (1970) *Adverse Reactions to Drugs*. London, Heinemann.

WALTON J.N. (1964) *Disorder of Voluntary Muscle*. London, Churchill.

WILKINS L. (1965) *Endocrine Disorders in Childhood and Adolescence*. Springfield, Charles C. Thomas.

Index